CBD: What You Need to Know

Second Edition

Other books by Gregory L. Smith, MD, MPH:

Medical Cannabis: Basic Science and Clinical Applications (OEM/Aylesbury Press, 2016)

THCV - The “Anti-Munchies Appetite Killer”

(Kindle Direct Publishing, 2019)

All titles available on Amazon.com.

Disclaimer:

The information provided in this book is current and vetted as of December 2019. New research is constantly coming out about *cannabis sativa* and cannabidiol (CBD), so the information contained in this book is subject to change and/or be amended with new research as it becomes available. This book is intended to give the reader a basic knowledge of CBD and its medical applications, as well as a broader framework of understanding upon which to build as more information becomes available.

Table of Content

Dedication:

To all those who have taken the time, energy, and oftentimes leaps of faith, to bring *cannabis sativa* out of its state of scientific suspended animation, and back into our medicine cabinets where it rightly belongs.

Thank you.

-Gregory L. Smith, MD, MPH

PREFACE: THE MEDICAL CANNABIS REFUGEE

A few years ago, I was invited to speak at a large medical cannabis convention in Boston about using cannabidiol (CBD) in treatment of a variety of conditions. After the lecture, I was invited to do a book signing. I love book signings, as they are an opportunity for me to interact on a personal level with the people who read my book.

One woman, a young mother of a daughter with epilepsy, came up to me to buy the book. She described the hardship of moving from North Carolina to Colorado to get medical marijuana for her daughter, who had intractable seizures. She said that she was able to get CBD oil in North Carolina by having it shipped legally to her home. However, her daughter's case of epilepsy only responded a little to the CBD-only oil.

She was able to get a small quantity of whole-plant medical marijuana that was very high in the ingredient CBD. She quickly found out that when she added this, her daughter's seizures all but disappeared, decreasing in frequency from dozens of times per week to once every month or so. She also found that rubbing pure THC oil inside her daughter's mouth right after a seizure helped her recover much more quickly from the negative aftereffects. Because whole-plant marijuana was a criminal offense in North Carolina, the family decided to move to Colorado, where they could get convenient and legal access to CBD, THC, and THCV.

This story is relevant in several ways; it shows that although CBD alone can be an excellent medication for many conditions, sometimes it is simply not enough, so doctors and patients should have access to all the beneficial compounds in marijuana -- not just CBD. The story also represents an opportunity to educate people about the many medical marijuana- related resources available. In each chapter of this book, I will provide some websites that I have found particularly useful to patients, family members and caregivers.

So, you want to learn about cannabidiol (CBD)?

You have probably heard about the exciting and novel medical benefits of marijuana, but perhaps you are concerned about the risk of getting "high" or "addicted" to THC, the psychoactive compound in whole-plant marijuana. Maybe you live in a state or country where marijuana (medical or otherwise) is regulated or not legal in its whole plant form per se, but you are able to legally access cannabidiol (CBD), and want to find out if it may be beneficial to you.

Perhaps yourself, a family member, or a loved one is currently suffering from one of the dozens of medical conditions— intractable epilepsy, anxiety, chronic pain, arthritis, or Multiple Sclerosis— that can respond to CBD, and want to learn more about how CBD works and how to use it. Or, perhaps you already have some preliminary knowledge of how CBD works, and simply want to achieve a deeper level of understanding of this wonderful compound.

You may have noticed that CBD oils and extracts are available without a prescription both in stores and online, and you may be wondering why a doctor's visit isn't generally required to get CBD. Unfortunately, over 95% of doctors or pharmacists have had no formal training on medical marijuana or CBD. That's why I decided to write this book; I felt it was time for the medical community to embrace this incredible plant. It is my hope that we soon learn to utilize it to its fullest potential, maximizing its benefits for the health and happiness of all.

About 15 years ago, I took a course on how to use marijuana medically for treatment of a variety of conditions. It occurred to me that there was no science-based textbook from which medical students and physicians could learn about medical marijuana. If a medical professional wanted to learn about medical marijuana, they had to painstakingly research each subject or condition, poring over studies and clinical anecdotes for small tidbits of info, some of which was rather outdated.

So, I spent two and a half years gathering the available research, including basic research in animals and tissue cultures, and clinical trials in humans. I synthesized this body of information into Medical Cannabis: Basic Science and Clinical Applications. This textbook came out in early 2016, and remains a bestseller among physicians, medical students, nurses, pharmacists and caregivers.

Strong resistance from physicians

Within a few months of publishing my textbook, I realized that most physicians and medical organizations, such as the American Medical Association, were still very much resistant to medical marijuana, feeling that there was not enough existing research to consider it as a 'serious' medication. Among my fellow physicians, there seemed to be a strong sense that medical marijuana legislation was just a means to bypass the prohibition against using marijuana for recreational purposes. This stubborn resistance to medical marijuana is changing, albeit slowly.

In the Spring of 2017, the National Academies of Sciences released a report entitled "The Health Effects of Cannabis and Cannabinoids: The Current State of Evidence and Recommendations for Research." This group of scientists and healthcare providers reviewed thousands of research studies, ultimately concluding that marijuana was effective as a treatment for several serious medical conditions and showed potential as a treatment for many others. Unfortunately, research has been significantly hindered by the federal government for the past 40 years.

Profit motivation from pharmaceutical companies

There is very little profit motivation amongst larger pharmaceutical companies to spend the millions of dollars necessary to get high-quality, marijuana-based pharmaceuticals approved by the FDA. The primary active ingredients of all marijuana-based medications will be THC and CBD, neither of which can be patented due to their organic nature and natural occurrence in the body. Any marijuana-based medication eligible for patent by a pharmaceutical company could be easily imitated by other companies without any patent infringement. Without patents, pharmaceutical companies would have a hard time making a profit from these medications.

Since 1999, the federal government has held a patent on all cannabinoids, including CBD, for their use as antioxidants and neuroprotectants. Litigation is still pending, however, and the FDA has yet to establish a clear policy on this issue of patent infringement with regards to cannabinoids.

The first FDA-approved drug made from cannabis extracts is Epidiolex®, an oral extract that costs $32,500 a year, and is approved for two rare forms of intractable childhood epilepsy. Smaller, more niche-based pharmaceutical companies, such as G.W. Pharmaceuticals from the U.K., have pharmaceuticals for sale in many countries, and are currently pending FDA approval of two drugs in the US. High-CBD hemp extracts (5-30% CBD) are generally not considered to be infringing on the Epidiolex® patent; however, I would defer to a lawyer to speak with authority on this matter.

Epidiolex® is 99.5% CBD extracted from a specific strain of medical marijuana. Very similar, 99.5% CBD extracts are available for about $100-$200 a month without a prescription. These extracts, available at dispensaries, health food stores, and online, are not covered by health insurance, because they are not specifically FDA-approved as Epidiolex® is, but they are readily available to patients and caregivers without a prescription.

Most FDA-approved pharmaceuticals are designed to be increasingly selective-- i.e., having a specific effect in one brain center or organ system in the body. However, CBD is exactly the opposite, having multiple effects on various receptors in the brain and body. In general, the higher the dose of CBD, the greater the number of target organ systems that will be impacted. Much research still needs to be done on the therapeutic benefits of CBD, dosing and balancing CBD with THC, and the 'entourage effect.' These concepts will be discussed in detail later in the book.

Patient Empowerment: How to educate your physician

Physicians are used to being in control of the patient-physician relationship and tend to be of the impression that they have all the answers to a patient's medical questions and concerns. This creates a significant problem when formulating a treatment plan with CBD, because 95% of physicians are taught nothing in medical school or residency about either THC or CBD and lack a basic understanding of the Endocannabinoid System (ECS).

While 5 FDA-approved cannabinoid medications are currently on the market, with several more in the later stages of clinical trials, the ECS and cannabinoids have traditionally not been taught in medical schools in the United States, due to a variety of sociopolitical and federal funding issues. This is changing rapidly, but it will probably be a few more years yet before a significant number of doctors and pharmacists have any legitimate working knowledge of medical cannabis or CBD.

A 2017 survey of the Association of American Medical Colleges (AAMC) Curriculum Inventory database revealed that only nine percent of curriculums contained any information on medical cannabis; eighty-four percent of doctors reported receiving no education on the topic in medical school or residency, and an equal number said that they felt unprepared to prescribed medical cannabis.[1] CBD is a remarkably safe compound, with a large therapeutic window and few contraindications, especially in contrast to most FDA-approved medications; still, physicians should be educated thoroughly on the endocannabinoid system (ECS) before prescribing CBD or other cannabinoid-based medications.

As the use of CBD is slowly filtering into the medical community, and small, profit-motivated pharmaceutical companies are moving ahead with high-cost medical marijuana preparations, I felt a strong need to write a concise, yet comprehensive book that will empower people to take hold of their right to have access to CBD-- a safe, legal, and effective medication.

Many people are under the impression they must visit a physician and be in a state-run marijuana registry to acquire CBD. Although laws vary state-to-state, in most states, neither a referral nor a prescription is required to legally obtain CBD products. This book will tell you how to make certain that you are purchasing safe, effective, and high-quality CBD products.

Laws are subject to change, and most lawmakers' current attitudes towards CBD (which are heavily influenced by financial incentives and lobbying from the pharmaceutical industry), may result in a crackdown on CBD products. When you do decide to purchase CBD, make sure to do some research beforehand to make certain that it is legal in your state or country.

The 2017 Institutes of Medicine report focused on medical cannabis, but also contained several findings specifically supportive of CBD for a variety of conditions. Some of the common conditions for which CBD can be a very effective treatment include chronic neuropathic pain from diabetes and HIV, radicular pain from degenerative disk disease, chronic myofascial pain, peripheral neuropathies such as CTS, local and diffuse arthritis, fibromyalgia, and anxiety.[2]

Based on animal studies, several dermatological conditions may be responsive to topical application of CBD, including psoriasis, eczema, Peyronie's disease, and Dupuytren's contractures.[3] In recent years, there has been an exponential increase in high-quality research and clinical trials on CBD and its therapeutic potential in the treatment of adult seizures, chronic neurodegenerative conditions, various forms of cancer, and inflammatory bowel diseases.[4] Presumably, as time goes on, even more previously undiscovered uses for CBD will come to light as the medical community continues to become more accepting and aware of this wondrous compound and all its potential

PART I: ALL ABOUT CBD

Chapter 1:
What Is Cannabidiol (CBD)?

Cannabidiol (CBD) is an oil found in the *cannabis sativa* plant. Unlike the other well-known ingredient of marijuana, tetrahydrocannabinol (THC), CBD is non-psychoactive, meaning that it doesn't result in the euphoric "high" that most people associate with smoking marijuana. CBD is especially prevalent in the flowers, or buds, of the plant. To a lesser degree, it is also prevalent in the stalks and leaves of the plant.

CBD is found in high concentrations in certain strains, while it is barely present in others. CBD is one of approximately 144 cannabinoid oils that can be found only in the cannabis plant. CBD, CBG (cannabigerol), and THC (tetrahydrocannabinol) are the three major cannabinoids found in large quantities in the cannabis plant, with many other minor cannabinoids such as CBDV (cannabivarin), THCV (tetrahydrocannabivarin), CBC (cannabichromine) existing in only trace amounts.

Because of their relatively low concentration in the marijuana plant, and due to numerous legal constraints on studying marijuana extracts, little research has yet been conducted on most of these minor cannabinoids. Over the next few years, we can expect a great deal more research on the potential therapeutic uses of these other cannabinoids.

Later in this chapter, you will find a list of many of the other lesser cannabinoids and their potential health benefits. This book is predominantly about CBD; However, before delving too deep into CBD and its uses, I will provide a more general introduction to medical cannabis in all its forms.

Hemp vs. Marijuana

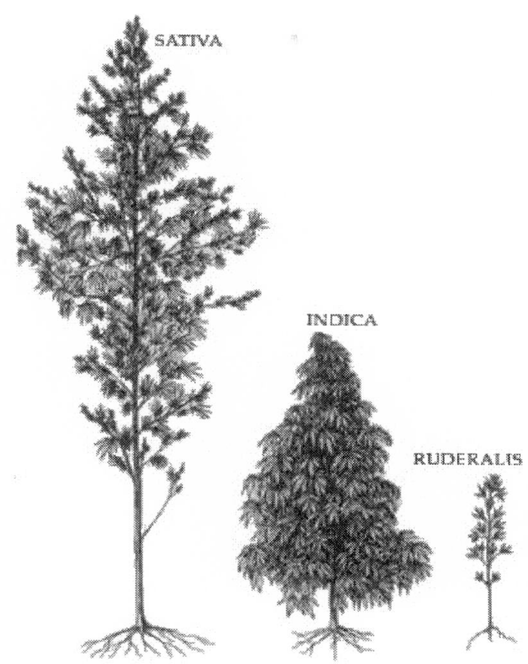

Historically, those strains of *cannabis sativa* that developed on the western side of the Himalayas after the end of the last ice age tended to grow into tall, thin plants with long, thin leaves. These strains, known as *cannabis sativa sativa*, developed an enzyme that resulted in the formation of predominantly CBD, with very little THC. Like THC, CBD is an odorless, tasteless chemical that is produced mostly in the flowering part of the female cannabis plant. This tall, thin, low-THC containing plant is the sub-genus of *cannabis sativa* commonly known as 'hemp'.

Those strains that developed on the colder, windier eastern side of the Himalayas tended to be short and bushy plants with broad, wide leaves. These strains developed a different enzyme that consequently produces THC and very little CBD; this sub-genus is known as *cannabis sativa indica.*

Even among those who are intimately involved with marijuana, there is still considerable confusion about the difference between 'marijuana' and 'hemp'. The terms 'hemp', and 'marijuana', both refer to the *cannabis sativa* plant.

However, several decades ago, it was arbitrarily decided by lawmakers that *cannabis sativa* containing less than 0.3% THC by weight ought to be classified as 'hemp', and strains containing more than 0.3% THC would constitute 'marijuana'.

Although insignificant from a scientific perspective, when it comes to their respective legality in the United States, the distinction between 'hemp' and 'marijuana' becomes crucial. When CBD oil is extracted from hemp plants (plants producing less than 0.3% THC), according to federal law, it is considered a "nutritional supplement"— legal and available over-the-counter in all 50 states; however, when the same CBD oil is extracted from 'marijuana' (*cannabis sativa* flowers containing more than 0.3% THC), it is classified as a Schedule I drug, with significant criminal consequences attributed to its use, production, and distribution.

In other words, the exact same oil can be treated either as an over-the-counter nutritional supplement, fully legal and available for purchase in all 50 states, or as a dangerous and illicit narcotic—scheduled along with heroin, cocaine and PCP--depending on subtle differences in classification of the plant it was sourced from. There is no legitimate medical or scientific reason for this, only the profit motivation of lawmakers and powerful pharmaceutical companies.

Hemp, in its raw form, has been used for millennia for a variety of applications: hemp fiber was used for fabric and rope, and hemp oil for nutritional and industrial purposes. Marijuana, in contrast, is used for the oils from the flower for medical or recreational purposes.

All cannabinoids, including CBD, are fat-soluble. The various formulations of CBD are of three types:

- **Full-spectrum CBD extracts** contain CBD, minor cannabinoids, terpenes, and 'significant' amounts of THC (>0.3%). Because they are above the legal threshold of THC content, these extracts are highly regulated and federally illegal.

- **Broad-spectrum CBD extracts** contain virtually no THC (< 0.3%), but they do contain all the naturally occurring terpenes and minor cannabinoids found in hemp oil, in addition to CBD.

- **CBD isolates** are distillates of pure (≥98%) CBD, containing no THC, minor cannabinoids, or terpenes.

Cannabinoid formulations are dosed and titrated in a manner that is entirely different from almost all other FDA-approved medications used by physicians. This has to do with how CBD interacts with receptors on cell membranes, which results in significant inter-individual variation in response to doses of CBD.[4] In addition, the specific metabolism and bioavailability of CBD from these formulations is highly variable due to fat solubility, gastric acid effects, rapid absorption into adipose tissue, and, perhaps most importantly, metabolism into inactive metabolites via the first-pass effect of the liver.[5]

There are several recent CBD formulations that use nanotechnology. Since CBD is highly biodegraded by the 'first-pass' effect of the liver after ingestion, tablets or capsules containing CBD or hemp oil would be mostly metabolized into inactive cannabinoid metabolites and excreted in the urine by the liver. However, in the past few years, various nanoparticle technologies have successfully been applied to CBD to make it more stable in the acid pH of the stomach so it is absorbed as a water-soluble preparation, missing this first-pass effect.[6] These nano-formulations are designed to be water-soluble and deliver more CBD into the bloodstream, but at the moment, there is little good research to confirm improved bioavailability or therapeutic benefit from these nanoparticle formulations.

Hemp Oil

Hemp oil is the oil that is extracted from non-euphoric hemp plants; it tends to be high in CBD, and very low in THC. CBD oil is hemp oil that has been further extracted and refined so that there are even higher levels of CBD in it. In the past two decades, several strains of hemp have been developed with increasingly higher concentrations of CBD, and even less THC.

The Charlotte's Web strain, developed in Colorado by the Stanley brothers for the treatment of intractable pediatric seizures, has a ratio of 20:1 CBD to THC, and less than 0.3% THC. There exist several other similar strains of high-CBD, very low-THC marijuana, but Charlotte's Web is among the most well-known and medically recognized.

Recreational strains of marijuana tend to have much higher amounts of THC than CBD. Since CBD mitigates the euphoric effects of getting high, only very small amounts of CBD are usually found in these recreational strains. The most popular recreational strains of marijuana are often 20% or more THC and 0.2% CBD, giving a ratio of 1:100 CBD to THC.

THC

This book is focused on CBD, so I will only briefly discuss THC here. Tetrahydrocannabinol (THC) is one of the two primary medically important cannabinoids found in high levels in marijuana, and the primary psychoactive cannabinoid in marijuana. It is also the primary component of marijuana that is associated with the most significant side effects; in extreme cases, bad reactions to THC can result in paranoia or even psychosis.

Still, THC has a wide array of medical effects that are much different from CBD, and when dosed properly, can be of great medical benefit. Using CBD in combination with THC in a 1:1 ratio greatly diminishes the euphoria associated with THC, thereby reducing the chance of developing an addiction or having an adverse reaction. A pure dose of 100-200 milligrams of a tincture or vaporizer of CBD can be given to someone experiencing an adverse reaction from recreational marijuana to rapidly decrease these negative effects.

Other Cannabinoids

There are about 144 different cannabinoids, so this list will just discuss those that are more medically important. All cannabinoids interact with receptors of the body's innate ECS to varying degrees, with varying medical and psychoactive effects. Because the names often sound similar, it can be helpful to refer to them by their abbreviations.

CBC (cannabichromene:)

No euphoric effects. May have anti-inflammatory and antiviral effects and help to facilitate pain relief; It also may have antidepressant effects.

CBG (cannabigerol:)

No euphoric effects. CBG may have anti-inflammatory effects, and may promote bone growth; it is currently being studied for its ability to inhibit tumor and cancer cell growth.

CBN (cannabinol:)

No euphoric effects. Similar to CBG, CBN may also promote bone growth and have anti-inflammatory effects. Currently being studied for treatment of insomnia.

THCV (tetrahydrocannabivarin:)

Shown to have significant health effects that vary notably from those of CBD. Among the properties of THCV are promoting fat loss, improving insulin resistance and blood sugar control, and improving blood lipids. In essence, THCV reverses the effects of the now-epidemic Metabolic Syndrome.

11-OH-THC (eleven hydroxytetrahydrocannabinol:)

Intense euphoric effects. This is not present in the plant, but when the liver metabolizes THC, it turns much of the THC into 11-OH-THC. It is considered the main active metabolite of THC after being consumed in an edible. It is more potent than THC, and crosses into the brain more easily than THC. It is associated with increased appetite.

Acidic forms of cannabinoids

All cannabinoids have an acidic carboxylated form, notated by the small letter ‘a’ after the abbreviation (e.g. THCa, CBDa and THCVa). The acidic forms are how the cannabinoids are naturally present in the raw plant material. After decarboxylation via heat or drying of the plant material, the acidic form is turned into the oxidized form, which behaves quite differently in the body; For example, THCa does not cause euphoria, and preliminary research suggests that it has many medical uses different from THC. The only way to get THCa or other acidic cannabinoids is to juice freshly harvested marijuana flowers and drink the fresh juice; if the juice is left for several days, it will naturally oxidize from THCa to THC.

Terpenes

In addition to the cannabinoids, there are several hundred terpenes that can be found in cannabis. Terpenes are the non-psychoactive organic compounds in cannabis; however, unlike cannabinoids, which are only found in marijuana, terpenes can be found in a wide variety of plants, herbs, fruits and vegetables. Terpenes are secreted in the same glands of the marijuana flower as cannabinoids, and they interact synergistically with cannabinoids as part of the entourage effect, which will be discussed in more detail later. Since THC and CBD are odorless, colorless, and tasteless, it is the terpenes and flavonoids in cannabis oil that give each different strain of marijuana its particular aroma and color.

Terpenes are only present in a small amount in the plant oils, but many of them have their own health effects. One in particular, beta caryophyllene, actually has health effects via one of the same receptors of the endocannabinoid system (ECS) that cannabinoids use. Beta caryophyllene is found in black pepper, hops, cloves and other plants.

There has not been much research yet on terpenes, but due to the known therapeutic potential of some, including beta caryophyllene, we may expect to see more research on terpenes in the future. All of the important terpenes are available individually, over-the-counter as nutritional supplements. Here are some of the more common ones.

Caryophyllene:

Smells like pepper or cloves; also found in black pepper, cloves and cotton. Unlike any other terpene, it binds to CB2 cannabinoid receptors in the body.

Limonene:

Smells like citrus; also found in fruit rinds, peppermint and juniper. Has antifungal and antibacterial effects.

Myrcene:

Smells like earthy cloves; also found in mango, hops and lemongrass. Has sedating, muscle-relaxing effects. Myrcene probably responsible for "in-the-couch" sensation.

Pinene:

Smells like pine needles; also found in pine, rosemary, basil, and parsley. Counteracts some adverse effects of THC.

Flavonoids

Flavonoids are also present in marijuana oils, as well as all fruits and vegetables. They have potent antioxidant effects; In addition, they also contribute to the aroma and color of the various cannabis strains.

Entourage effect

Whole-plant marijuana oil is made up of a combination of THC, CBD, other minor cannabinoids, and a wide array of terpenes and flavonoids. Research in the 1980s with pure, synthetic THC analogues, without any other cannabinoids or terpenes, has shown that THC works more effectively and with far fewer side effects when CBD and terpenes are present. This synergistic and modifying effect is known as the 'entourage effect'.

The entourage effect is an important consideration in the development of cannabis-based medications. Often, the medications will be shown by the ratio of CBD to THC; for example, the best tinctures for childhood seizures are around between 18:1, a very high CBD to THC ratio. Pain is usually best treated with 1:1 medication.

How is CBD Extracted?

The oils in cannabis, including cannabinoids and terpenes, have been extracted via various methods for over a hundred years. The extracted oils are then further processed to increase the percentage of all or specific cannabinoids. A wide variety of solvents are used to dissolve the oils in the plant material, and the type of extraction methodology will determine what contaminants are in the extract.

Repeated extraction techniques result in less and less residual plant material, and consequently a lighter and clearer fluid. Different extraction techniques can absorb different oils from the plant more or less effectively. Olive oil, and ethanol usually extract more of the terpenes than the other solvents.

Hydrocarbon Solvents

Various hydrocarbons, including benzene, butane, hexane, and propane, can be used to dissolve the oil into a liquid. A slight remnant of these solvents usually remains in the extract. Since these hydrocarbons sometimes contain carcinogens, especially after heating, extracts made using these solvents are not recommended.

Ingestible Solvents

Several ingestible solvents, such as ethanol, olive oil, coconut oil, and butter can be used to dissolve the cannabinoids into an edible liquid. These solvents are safe, and, of course, edible; however, food-grade oils are also perishable. These extracts are generally made for ingestion as an extract, or in cannabis butter for making edibles.

Carbon Dioxide

Either supercritical or subcritical carbon dioxide (CO2) extraction is currently the safest and most popular means of obtaining high-purity extracts. The oil that is extracted via carbon dioxide is very high in purity and is free from chlorophyll and most other plant contaminants.

CO_2 is used under high pressure and at extremely low temperatures to isolate the medicinal oils from the contaminants that are often present with other extraction methodologies. Therefore, the CO_2 extraction process is ideal for an extract that is to be inhaled or ingested.

Chapter 2:
History and Legality

Throughout human history, innumerable plants have been discovered to have euphoric or medicinal effects. The earliest medications that our ancestors used were from plants: opium for pain relief, foxglove and digitalis, willow bark and aspirin, cinchonine and quinine. Marijuana, with its potent aroma and rapid onset of effects, was quickly determined by our ancient ancestors to have medicinal value.

Cannabis sativa grows naturally in many tropical parts of the world, and has been used for its fiber and oil-bearing seeds for 11,000 years-- almost as long a time as hunter-gatherers have been planting grain and domesticating animals. Marijuana plants were made into fiber for cloth and rope, and the oil from the flower and seeds was utilized for a variety of household applications.

Ancient use of marijuana

The first recorded medical use of marijuana was described in Indochinese medical texts more than 5,000 years ago. It was already known to be useful for a variety of physical and mental conditions. A Chinese medical text of the time prescribed marijuana leaves for tapeworm; the seeds were also pulverized and added to wine to help with constipation and hair loss.

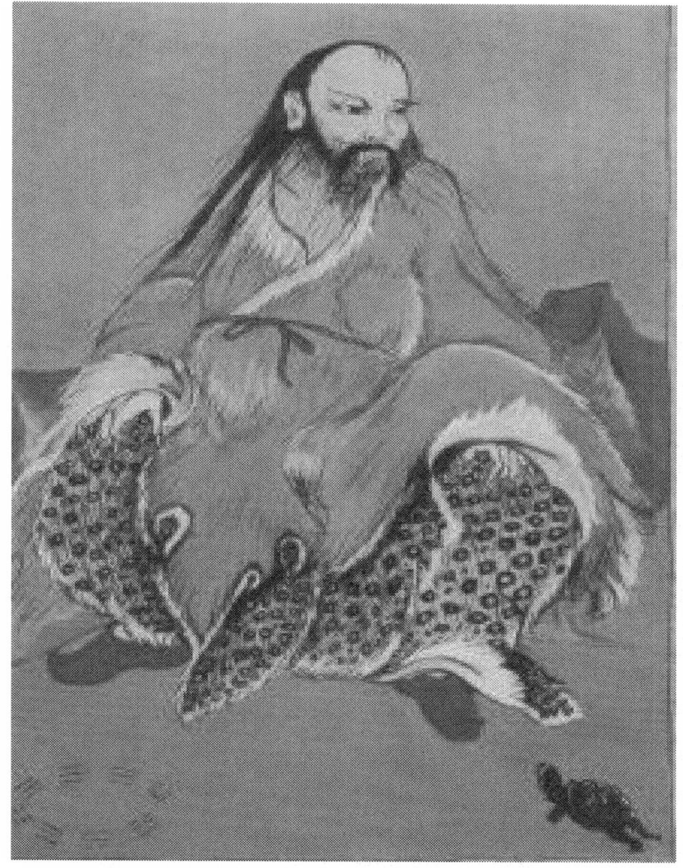

Chinese Emperor FU HSI (2900 BC) recommended medical cannabis

Marijuana use, for both recreational and medicinal purposes, spread quickly throughout the Greek and Roman empires, and subsequently throughout the Islamic empire. In 440 B.C.E., Herodotus discussed the Scythians using cannabis to make a vapor for steam baths. By the Middle Ages, it was regularly being used externally as a balm for muscle and joint pain.

Cannabis was introduced to the Americas by the Spaniards in 1545 for use as fiber; hemp became the first major fiber-producing plant in the US. By 1619, King James I ordered every colonist to grow 100 plants specifically for export. By the end of the 18th century, hemp was a major crop throughout the Americas.

Western medical use of marijuana

Although the plants were already ubiquitous throughout the US, marijuana did not make its way into Western medicine until 1839. At that time, Dr. William B. O'Shaughnessy returned from India with considerable experience using marijuana for medical purposes. He encouraged physicians to recommend it for insomnia, pain, muscle spasms and other physical conditions, and cannabis soon became an accepted medical treatment.

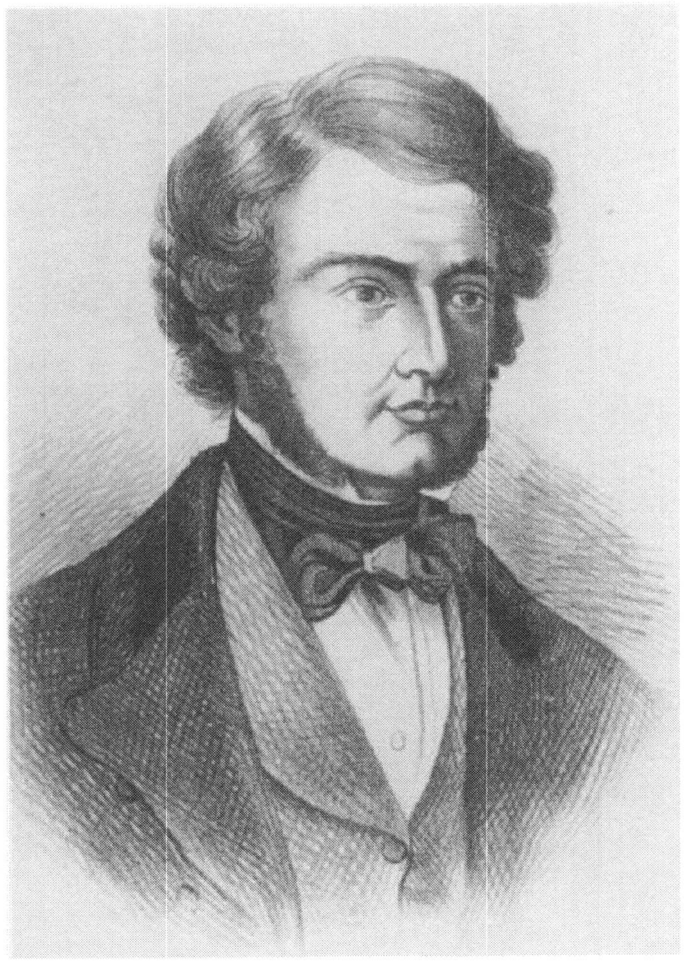

William Brooke O'Shaughnessy, 1809-1889

After its introduction and widespread acceptance into medical practice of the time, it started to be used for a wide variety of ailments, including gonorrhea, cholera, whooping cough and asthma, predominantly in the form of an orally ingested tincture. It is said that Queen Victoria used cannabis tincture for menstrual cramps.

Cannabis Indica Tincture

The potency, efficacy and side effects of various medicinal preparations of marijuana extracts vary significantly. For decades, these tinctures were sold as "patent medicines", and therefore the ingredients were secret. By the late 19th century, laws were already being enacted to address issues with mislabeling, adulteration, and sale of "poisons."' In addition, recreational marijuana usage in upscale hashish parlors flourished next to the thriving opium dens of the late 19th century.

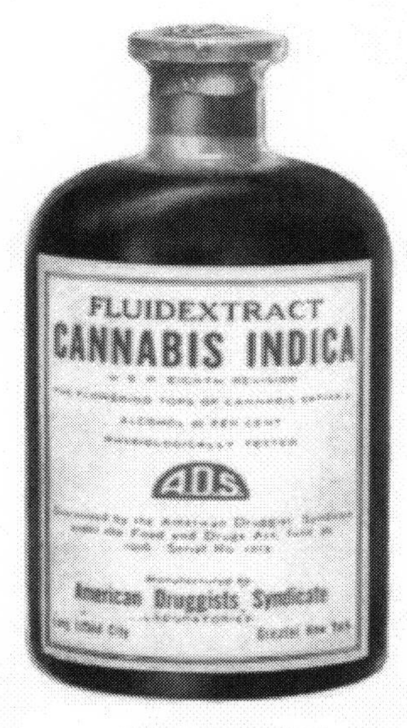

By the beginning of the 20th century, laws in several states required prescriptions for marijuana extracts. By this time, cannabis was the second most common ingredient in medications, and there existed over 2000 cannabis-containing preparations from over 280 manufacturers.

US Marijuana Laws

The Pure Food and Drug Act of 1906 and several state laws were passed to restrict "habit-forming drugs." These were the start of a series of laws to control and regulate drugs. In addition, after over a decade of alcohol prohibition, smoking cannabis, which had previously been associated with Mexican migrant workers and black jazz musicians, was gaining popularity for the first time among the general public.

This resulted in an immediate backlash from the federal government, who began utilizing the term 'marijuana', a slang term meaning "Mary Jane" in Spanish, on all government documents. The intention of this move was to vilify the drug and its users, separating smoked marijuana from the very popular *cannabis sativa* elixirs that were being used medicinally. The 1937 film *Reefer Madness* is a classic example of the propaganda of this time.

ADULTS ONLY!
The Sweet PILL that MAKES LIFE BITTER!
WOMEN CRY FOR IT- MEN DIE FOR IT!
"REEFER MADNESS"
SEE
DRUG-CRAZED ABANDON

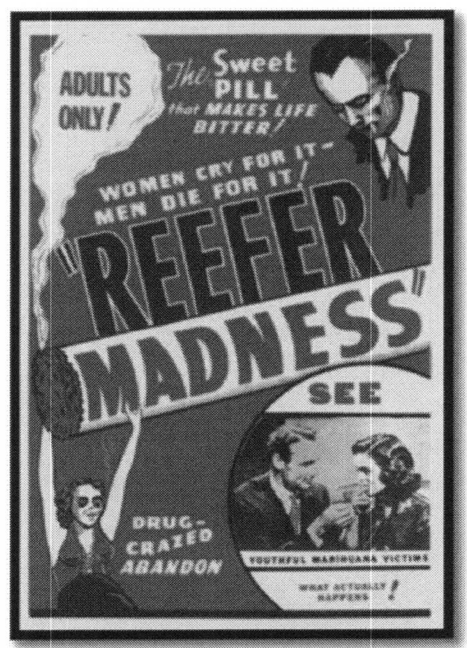

At the same time, the Marijuana Tax Act of 1937 imposed a levy of one dollar per ounce on marijuana used for medical use, and $100 per ounce for recreational use. This law effectively made non-medical or non-industrial use, possession, or sale of marijuana illegal throughout the US.

At that time, the fledgling American Medical Association (AMA) was opposed to this law, and correctly thought that it would impede future research into the drug. By 1938, the Federal Pure Food, Drug and Cosmetics Act established the framework that we still use today to regulate prescription and non-prescription drugs. By 1951, the Boggs Act added *cannabis sativa* to the list of narcotic drugs.

The use of marijuana for medicinal purposes dramatically decreased over the course of the early twentieth century. There was some research in the 50's and 60's for its potential as a treatment for glaucoma, but far superior ophthalmic medications became available.

The molecule THC was not differentiated from *cannabis sativa* until Dr. Raphael Mechoulam discovered it in Israel in 1964 (CBD had already been isolated, as early as 1940.) In the 1970's, a synthetic version of THC called Marinol® was approved by the FDA for chemotherapy-induced nausea and vomiting, and later, for cancer and AIDS-related wasting syndrome. The intense euphoric side effects from pure THC, and necessity of swallowing oral capsules while nauseous, made this a poor clinical choice. The advent of superior medications has made these synthetic cannabinoid pharmaceuticals obsolete from their original, FDA-approved indications.

In 1969, during a very turbulent period of anti-war social unrest, President Nixon pushed for a comprehensive crackdown on drug use, or what he called a 'war on drugs.' He was especially focused on marijuana because of its association with the anti-war movement. The Controlled Substances Act (CSA) was passed as part of the Comprehensive Drug Abuse Prevention and Control Act of 1970; This legislation made the possession or distribution of *cannabis sativa* criminal at a federal level and created the five Schedules of Dangerous Drugs. The Drug Enforcement Administration (DEA), together with the FDA, placed *Cannabis sativa* into Schedule I, where the drug was determined to have "no medical use" and come with "high risk of addiction." This legislation effectively put an end to all serious scientific study of medical marijuana, including CBD, and severely limited the study of other cannabinoids.

CBD research

In the early 1990s, the Endocannabinoid System (ECS) was discovered. We learned that cannabinoids have their effects in the body by binding to natural cannabinoid receptors in the brain and body that make up the ECS. Since this natural system in our body was discovered, researchers have conducted tens of thousands of studies in animal models and tissue culture on the effects of the various cannabinoids; However, the main research on CBD in humans has been done by GW Pharmaceuticals in trials for children with rare intractable epilepsy. CBD is one of the three cannabinoids present in high quantities in marijuana, and a growing body of research has shown how CBD can have a wide array of beneficial medical effects.

Over the decades since phytocannabinoids were found to mimic the effects of our natural endocannabinoids, most of the attention and research has gone towards THC. With rapid and obvious psychomotor effects, as well as other relatively obvious effects on nausea, appetite, and pain, THC has been the darling of pharmacologic research among cannabinoid medications. This trend has changed in the past decade or so with much greater awareness of the importance of CBD, as well as the ratio of CBD to THC in medical cannabis formulations.

Along with the notorious side effect of "the munchies", THC is associated with almost all adverse effects of cannabinoid medications, including euphoria, addiction, psychosis, anxiety, agitation, and dysphoria. CBD, on the other hand, has been shown to have many more medical effects than THC, with a much broader therapeutic window and safety profile.

US Medical Marijuana Laws

After several failed attempts, California was the first state to pass Proposition 215 in 1996, known as the Compassionate Care Act. This, along with the passing of Senate Bill 420 in 2003, allowed for the networking of growers, caregivers, and healthcare providers, and an identification card system for medical marijuana. As of the time of this writing, 42 states and the District of Columbia have passed some sort of legalized medical cannabis laws.

Whole-plant vs. CBD-only laws

Whole-plant marijuana refers to strains of cannabis flower that contain measurable quantities of THC (≥ 0.3% by dry weight), so there may be euphoric effects associated with its use. Many states allow for CBD-only strains, which means the plant or extract must be very low (<0.3%) in THC, but higher in CBD; Charlotte's Web is a classic example of such a strain.

The regulations and requirements on medical cannabis vary considerably across state and country lines, so great care ought to be taken when reviewing laws to find out if they apply to your own state. New York state, for example, allows for medical marijuana to be administered in any number of forms, but specifically forbids the smoking of cannabis flower.

Some states only allow medical marijuana for certain Qualified Conditions (QC), such as Multiple Sclerosis or Alzheimer's disease. These QC vary considerably from state to state and are often based solely on political motives. That said, the generally recognized medical efficacy of THC and CBD and the innate safety of these drugs has underpinned the support and continued expansion of medical marijuana laws in the US and around the world.

Changes to Federal Marijuana Policy

In 2009, based on the rapidly evolving changes at the state level in legalization of medical cannabis, the US Attorney General stated, "It will not be a priority to use federal resources to prosecute patients with serious illnesses or their caregivers who are complying with state laws on medical marijuana, but we will not tolerate drug traffickers who hide behind claims of compliance with state law to mask activities that are clearly illegal.»

In December 2014, Congress and the Obama Administration quietly put an end to the federal prohibition against medical cannabis as a tiny part of a federal spending bill. However, federal banking laws still force medical dispensaries to operate as "cash only" businesses.

Most recently, the prescription opioid epidemic that has been ravaging the US has helped to push cannabis back into the spotlight as a much safer and less addictive alternative to opioids for pain control. Cannabis has been shown to be very helpful with transitioning patients off opioids, a point which I will be discussing in depth in a later chapter.

The FDA continues to list *cannabis sativa* as a Schedule I drug, but major efforts are currently underway to re-schedule it to a lower drug classification, or perhaps de-schedule marijuana as a drug altogether, and instead treat it as a regulated substance, such as alcohol or tobacco.

US CBD laws

CBD that originates in *cannabis sativa* (≥ 0.3% THC) is still considered to be an illegal drug, and any extracts from the plant are still an illegal drug at a federal level in the US. Using THC requires a doctor's recommendation letter in those states where it is legal; However, Epidiolex®, a 99.5% CBD extract in sesame oil, is FDA-approved, and available by prescription in all 50 states.

Unfortunately, it is only FDA-approved for oral use, which means it must be ingested. This route of administration results in over 90% of the CBD being metabolized by the liver to inactive metabolites, so the dose of Epidiolex® is 1600mg a day for an average adult, at a cost of $32,500 a year. Artisanal CBD extracts, in contrast, are recommended to be taken sublingually, where they are absorbed directly into the bloodstream, avoiding the first-pass effect of the liver and resulting in the need to use only a fraction of the dose (50-100mg a day), at a tiny fraction of the cost of Epidiolex®.

In December 2018, President Donald Trump signed the federal Farm Bill of 2018 into law. This law defined hemp as distinct from marijuana and essentially ended prohibition of the cultivation, distribution, manufacturing and sale of all hemp-related products, including hemp oil extracts. This has led to a plethora of high-quality, US-grown hemp oil.

The 2018 Farm Bill has clarified many of the issues related to the use, sale, and intrastate transportation of hemp-based products. As a result of the new law, the Drug Enforcement Agency (DEA) has removed hemp and hemp products from its purview under the Controlled Substance Agency (CSA), and the FDA is now responsible for hemp products for human consumption. This has resulted in significant improvements in the manufacturing, labeling, regulation, and quality of these products.

Prior to the new law, there were hundreds of hemp products available for human consumption, often manufactured with inadequate quality, safety, and labeling, and not always laboratory tested for contaminants or potency.[7, 8]

Until the passage of the Farm Bill, there was little assurance that the hemp and CBD formulations being marketed as "pure" CBD products were free of contaminants -- or that they contained any CBD whatsoever, for that matter.

The net result of these changes has been wide and popular acceptance of over-the-counter CBD products, as well as easy accessibility of a wide array of CBD formulations. In fact, use of CBD products is expected to triple by 2022.[9] Healthcare providers are becoming increasingly aware and cooperative with the fact that their patients are supplementing with CBD and other hemp-based formulations as adjunct treatments for their conditions.

CBD laws in other countries

In most countries, pure CBD or low-THC hemp oil (<0.3%) is not considered a scheduled substance or illicit drug; much more commonly, it is categorized as a "cosmetic ingredient" or "nutritional supplement". In some places, however, hemp is still a controlled substance. It is generally a good idea to check individual import laws and requirements by country before traveling abroad with any CBD or hemp products, even if the traveler is a medical patient and the product in question falls under the <0.3% threshold for THC content.

Epidiolex®

An UK-based pharmaceutical company has been developing several marijuana-based prescription medications over the past 20 years. One of these medications, Epidiolex®, a 99.5% CBD formulation extracted from the flowers of a specific strain of *cannabis sativa*, was given an "orphan drug" designation by the FDA for the treatment of two very rare forms of childhood intractable seizures. Epidiolex®, approved by the FDA in late 2018, is available at pharmacies around the US and may be covered by some health insurance providers.

This granting of "prescription drug" status to CBD (it is currently on Schedule

V of the Controlled Substances Act) has created great concern among the manufacturers of artisanal CBD extracts, who may now have to stop selling or producing their products if they are found to be causing patent infringement or other legal issues with the manufacturers of Epidiolex®. Interested readers can research Epidiolex® to learn more.

Artisanal CBD Formulations

Other than Epidiolex®, which is a 99.5% isolate of CBD and is available at pharmacies, there are dozens of manufacturers around North America that manufacture artisanal CBD formulations. (I use the term 'artisanal' here to describe all these non-FDA cannabinoid formulations.) These artisanal formulations are available at health food stores, online, and even at gas stations and minimarts; many large pharmacy chains are now offering their own artisanal CBD formulations over-the-counter.

These formulations are manufactured by using CBD isolate (≥98%) and adding a vehicle such as coconut or sesame seed oil (similar to Epidiolex®). These isolate-based formulations contain none of the other important terpenes or minor cannabinoids found in hemp oil. Research suggests that terpenes and minor cannabinoids help CBD to work more effectively at the receptors, and move the dose-response curve to the left, thereby reducing necessary doses via the 'entourage effect'.[10]

The other category of CBD formulations, known as 'broad-spectrum' or 'whole plant' extracts, are made by distilling and extracting the hemp oil so that there are high levels of CBD in the formulation (typically, less than 20% CBD). The remaining portion is the whole plant hemp oil, which is a wonderful combination of minor cannabinoids, terpenes, and often chlorophyll.

Isolates are generally much less expensive than broad-spectrum extracts, making these CBD-based products deceptively attractive to doctors and patients. Broad-spectrum products are preferable, however, as they have been shown to have superior dose-response curves due to the 'entourage effect' mentioned above.

The net result of poor-quality, inexpensive products, often made with isolates of CBD from China, can mean inaccurate doses and oftentimes, contamination. Therefore, depending on its relative quality, the usage of a CBD isolate may show little or no therapeutic benefit. If the medication doesn't do what it is supposed to, a patient who might otherwise have been a good candidate for treatment with CBD may be put off from it due to lack of access to quality products.

Another issue that can arise is if the doctor recommending the CBD is not well-versed in the pharmacokinetics (PK) and pharmacodynamics (PD) of CBD, i.e. absorption and metabolism, and how much CBD gets into the bloodstream (bioavailability).

For example, if CBD is ingested (swallowed into the stomach) and not absorbed by inhalation or under the tongue, a whopping 90% of the compound is turned into inactive metabolites via the 'first-pass effect' of the liver.[11] Therefore, only a tiny fraction of the ingested dose of CBD will eventually become bioavailable in the blood for therapeutic effects.

Cannabinoids, including CBD, are lipid-soluble, unlike the majority of medications which are water-soluble. Therefore, the absorption and stability of the formulation is impacted by stomach acid and food content. Due to these factors, it is vital that the provider chooses the proper dose, route and method of administration of CBD.

Another factor that can impede absorption of a CBD product is the use of enteric-coated capsules, which often do not break down in time for the CBD to be released and absorbed into the bloodstream. A recent study showed that half of all patients who ingested enteric coated capsules of CBD had zero absorption of the CBD inside the capsule.

Physician education and cannabinoids

It is estimated that only about one percent of physicians in the US regularly recommend medical marijuana in their practice, and only about five percent have had any education on the ECS or training on the use of cannabinoids such as THC and CBD.[12] Although marijuana has a long and respected history as a medicine, it was not until the early 1990's that the ECS was discovered and researchers began to evaluate how cannabinoids work in the brain and body, by which point most of today's practicing physicians were already out of medical school. Not unexpectedly, there is essentially no consistent training or education of medical students, even to this day, on cannabinoids, medical marijuana, or the ECS.

The first medical marijuana law passed in California in 1996, and the dominant stance of the medical community at the time was that such legal provisions were simply loopholes by which potheads could bypass the prohibition against the recreational use of marijuana. This is slowly beginning to change, but to date, almost all the existing research on medical cannabi for humans is either very outdated (from the 70's or 80's), poor in quality, or pertaining to synthetic pharmaceuticals, not whole-plant marijuana.

Only in the past few years have high-quality, whole-plant marijuana studies in humans begun to emerge as legalization efforts push forward. Now, however, physicians are beginning to understand the incredible therapeutic potential of cannabis and cannabinoid-based medication for a wide array of conditions. It is my hope that this trend continues as more research becomes available.

Chapter 3:
How Does CBD Work?

CBD is very safe and effective at treating a wide variety of conditions with very few adverse reactions. CBD is responsible for about 80% of the medical effects of marijuana. Unlike THC, there is no euphoria associated with CBD, and no concern about addiction or dependency. In general, CBD can be considered an adjunct, or helper, to be used in conjunction with other medications that are already available. In the future, CBD may be considered a preventive medicine, and taken in a small, once-a-day dose to prevent or slow the progress of a wide array of chronic degenerative conditions.

Endocannabinoid System (ECS)

Like THC and other cannabinoids, CBD works by impacting the body's endocannabinoid system (ECS). The ECS is a natural system in our brain and body that is present in all animals and fish, evolutionarily dating back some 600 million years. The ECS's job is to modulate other systems in the body that can become overheated or stressed. It is like a braking system that can "slow down" a wide variety of systems in the body, including pain perception, gastrointestinal motility, memory, sleep, response to stress, pain and appetite, to name a few.

The ECS has unique functions throughout the body, but especially in the brain and the immune system; in fact, ECS receptors are the most common receptors in the brain and the second most common receptors in the body, showing exactly how important is the ECS. There are ECS receptors in every organ system in the body to help maintain the organ system in homeostasis or balance.

Nerve cells, called neurons, release chemical messengers called neurotransmitters. There are literally hundreds of different types of neurotransmitters released in the body depending on what system is involved.

When there are too many chemical messengers being released, and a specific system in getting out of control, the ECS releases, on demand, its own specific chemical messengers to slow down the release of these chemical messengers.

In this way, the ECS keeps several of the body's systems in balance. The ECS uses two different chemicals, anandamide (ANA) and 2-arachidonoylglycerol (2-AG.) These two chemicals are called *endocannabinoids*, or the innate cannabinoids made by the body naturally. These endocannabinoids work by attaching to a cannabinoid receptor on the cell. THC and CBD work by imitating the body's naturally occurring endocannabinoids.

There are two ECS receptors that we know of, that are named simply cannabinoid receptor 1 (CB1) and cannabinoid receptor 2 (CB2.) There are probably a few more, but they have not been discovered yet. Some systems in our brain and body have CB1 receptors, some have CB2, and some have both.

Much as a lock can only be opened once the key is put in, the 'lock' is the cannabinoid receptor on the cell membrane, and the 'key' is the endocannabinoid chemical, ANA or 2-AG. Once the endocannabinoid is released, it is quickly broken down by enzymes in the area, so that the effect is only short-lived, maybe milliseconds.

The ECS was discovered as recently as the 1990s. We have natural endocannabinoids that can become depleted in response to chronic perceived stress, and oxidative stress from the modern stressful lifestyle, the inflammatory modern diet and environmental toxins[3, 4, 5, 6]. There is growing evidence that a number of common conditions are due to endocannabinoid deficiency. These Clinical Endocannabinoid Deficiency Syndromes (CEDS) include migraine, irritable bowel syndrome, fibromyalgia and possibly anxiety [7, 8, 9,].

Plant cannabinoids are known as phytocannabinoids, or just cannabinoids. They mimic the effects of the body's endocannabinoids. The phytocannabinoids work by mimicking natural endocannabinoids at the cannabinoid receptors, and therefore, are postulated to make up for the innate deficiencies.

Endocannabinoid receptors

Once inhaled or ingested, these plant-based cannabinoids are absorbed into the bloodstream and travel all over the brain and body. These cannabinoids then bind to CB1 and CB2 receptors in the brain and certain organs in the body just as do ANA and 2-AG. This results in similar effects to the body's endocannabinoid chemicals, 2-AG and ANA.

When we use medical marijuana, we can have much higher doses of cannabinoids than our body is able to make on its own, thus resulting a medical or therapeutic effect. There are no specific enzymes in the body to immediately break down the cannabinoids from marijuana, so the effects last much longer than with the naturally occurring endocannabinoids.

Different cannabinoids in marijuana interact directly or indirectly with the CB1 and CB2 receptors; the way in which the cannabinoids interact with these receptors determines which medical effects and what adverse side effects we can expect. Sometimes the cannabinoids stimulate the CB1 and/ or CB2 receptors, sometimes they have the opposite effects of stimulation, called antagonism, and sometimes the cannabinoids just sit on the receptor and block the natural endocannabinoids from stimulating the receptor.

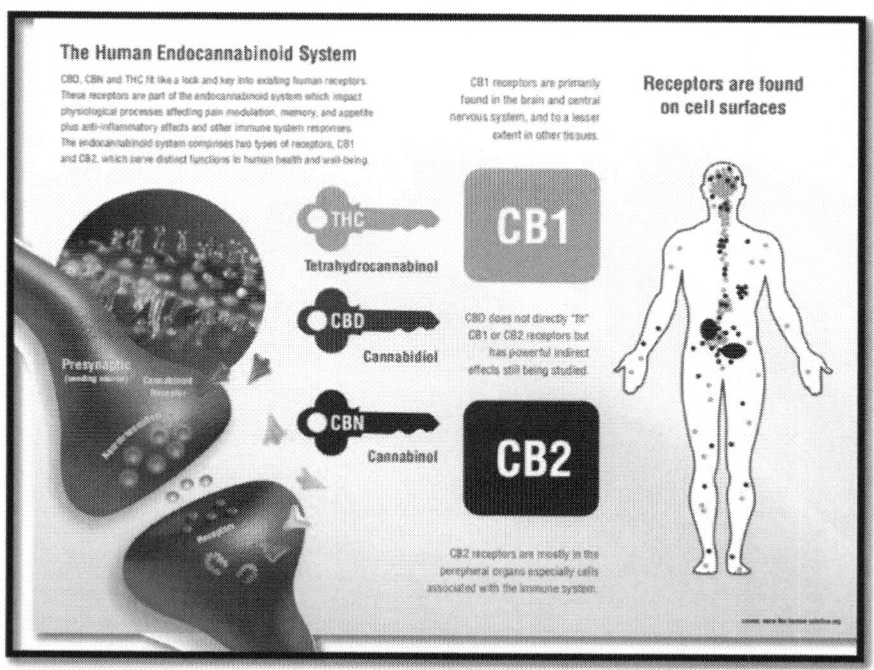

In general, CBD does not directly interact with the CB1 or CB2 receptors, but instead blocks an important enzyme that breaks down our natural cannabinoid ANA. It also occupies the proteins that transport endocannabinoids. So, the net result of both of these effects is that CBD results in an increase of our naturally occurring endocannabinoids, throughout the brain and body. This can be thought of as increasing our cannabinoid tone.

Cannabinoid tone

Cannabinoid tone is an important concept for determining likelihood that CBD may work therapeutically.[32] The ECS is involved with maintaining homeostasis in every organ system in the body, constantly active throughout the various centers of the brain and immune system. The number and type of receptors is also highly variable throughout the body; for example, the lack of measurable quantities of cannabinoid receptors in the brainstem is one of the reasons that it is essentially impossible to overdose of cannabis. Our heart and lung drivers originate in the brainstem, and ECS does not have any receptors there to result in respiratory or cardiac failure.

One of the goals of cannabinoid medications is to change the cannabinoid tone selectively, depending on which condition we are treating. The ECS releases endocannabinoids (ANA and 2-AG) only on-demand and local to wherever they are needed to slow down neural messaging. However, when we give someone cannabinoid medication, it enters the blood through the lungs or liver, flooding the entire body's ECS with significant amounts of CBD. There are even specific transport systems on the blood-brain barrier that rapidly move cannabinoid medications into the brain.[33] So, we need to dose the patient based on what part of the ECS we want to impact, and how much.

There are two types of cannabinoid tone, static and dynamic tone. The level of static tone is probably genetically determined, and may have an impact our personality and mood throughout our life.[6] The static tone of the ECS activity occurs without the need for endocannabinoids. The dynamic tone is the marked increase in ECS activity that occurs in response to endocannabinoids or phytocannabinoids.[32, 34]

CB1 receptors

The CB1 receptors are found in certain brain centers and in every organ system in the body. Here is a list of most of the brain centers and their associated function:

- **Hippocampus** - Learning, memory, stress related to adverse memories
- **Hypothalamus** - Appetite
- **Limbic System** - Anxiety
- **Cerebral Cortex** - Pain processing, higher cognitive functions
- **Prefrontal Cortex** - Reward and Addiction
- **Basal Ganglia** - Sleep, movement
- **Medulla** - Nausea and vomiting chemoreceptor

All organ systems in the body have CB1 receptors, including the uterus, cardiovascular system, adipose tissue, gastrointestinal tract, pancreas, bone and liver. We are still learning exactly how the ECS modulates these organs.

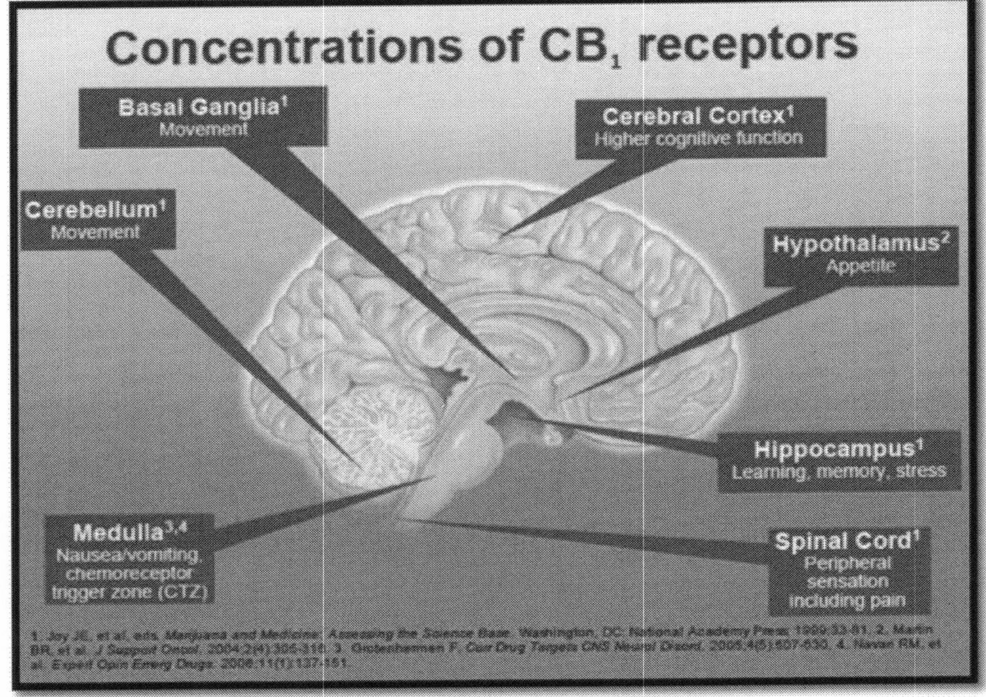

(graphic from theleafonline.com)

CB2 receptors

The CB2 receptors are found mostly in the immune system cells in the brain and body. These cells are involved with immunity and inflammation. The cells with CB2 receptors include monocytes, macrophages, B-cells, T-cells, and thymus gland cells. These have to do with modulating the release of chemicals involved with inflammation, swelling, immune response, cell migration and programmed cell death. In general, when the CB2 receptors are activated, the immune or inflammatory response is turned down.

CB2 receptors are also found in our bone's osteoblast cells. These cells work in tandem with osteoclasts to create new healthy bone cells. Studies have shown that activation of CB2 receptors results in improved healing of fractures and reduces osteoporosis.

Many tissues or organs of the body have both CB1 and CB2 receptors, providing different, often counter-balancing functions. Some of these include skin, brain, liver, and bone.

When tissues are injured, even if they usually don't have CB2 receptors, they will up-regulate CB2 receptors in the cell membranes in response to the injury in order to help control the amount of inflammation during the post-injury phase.

TRPV1 - Capsaicin receptor

Another receptor that responds cannabinoids is called transient receptor potential vanilloid 1 (abbreviated TRPV1). This is often called the 'capsaicin receptor.'[15] Capsaicin, a common ingredient in topical muscle balms, is the hot, irritating compound in chili peppers. TRPV1 is found mostly in the skin, although the receptors are found throughout the body and in the brain to a much lesser degree. TRPV1 is responsible for detecting and regulating body temperature and creating the sensation of pain in reaction to severe heat.

CBD, acetaminophen, hot temperatures, and several other chemicals activate TRPV1 receptors, initially sending heat sensations to the brain. However, with prolonged or intense activation, this leads to the receptors becoming desensitized, leading to a decrease in TRPV1-mediated release of inflammatory substances, and consequently pain reduction.

OTC topical creams with low concentrations (0.025-0.075%) of capsaicin probably act by counter-irritant effects, similar to camphor, and menthol._

Altering Cannabinoid Tone

In addition to using CBD to change of cannabinoid tone, we can change several lifestyle factors to increase our cannabinoid tone and improve our health.

Microbiome: There is increasing evidence that the bacteria in our colon, known as the microbiome, is a major regulator of the ECS. People should avoid unnecessary antibiotics, as these damage the natural microbiome balance in the gut. Also try pro- and prebiotics to get that promote healthy colon bacteria in the biome.

Anti-Inflammatory Diet: Pro-inflammatory foods, such as dairy products, processed meat, fried foods with trans-fats, or too many calories in general are bad for the ECS, by promoting oxidative stress in our body and brain.

Exercise: Sedentary behavior is harmful to the ECS, and exercise is essential to improving tone. A low-stress, low-impact aerobic program is recommended.

Genetics: ECS dysfunction has some genetic tendencies, so be extra careful if there are others in your family who have chronic migraine, fibromyalgia, chronic depression, or an autoimmune disease. Pay attention and be mindful about any unhealthy habits you may share.

Reduce stress and insomnia: The ECS maintains balance, and a body that is stressed out and unrested can lead to imbalance in the ECS tone. Mindfulness training, yoga, tai chi and other forms of meditation lead to improvement of balance and improved cannabinoid tone.

Change in number of receptors

ECS receptors are shaped like little buttons on the membrane. The number or density of these receptors on the outside of the cell membrane determines by how often the receptors are activated. Over time, if there is excessive stimulation of these receptors, then the number of receptors on the cell membrane will tend to decrease, this is called down-regulation. Therefore, it will take more of the cannabinoid to get the same effect. If there is not enough stimulation of these receptors, over time, the number of receptors will tend to increase, this is called up-regulation. This will result in more effects from lower doses of cannabinoids.

In order to learn how to dose CBD effectively, it is important to understand the importance of finding just the right dose that does not result in up- or down-regulation of the receptors on the cell membranes.

THC

When THC binds to the receptors, it only partially opens the lock. This is called being a partial agonist. THC binds to both CB1 and CB2 receptors. The euphoric effects of THC are due to the CB1 binding in certain brain centers. THC is one of the few well-studied cannabinoids that has consistent binding on CB1 receptors.

CBD

CBD works via the ECS, but unlike THC, it does not directly bind to CB1 or CB2 receptors. Instead, it indirectly increases the activity of CB2 receptors by blocking a certain enzyme known as FAAH. By blocking this enzyme, there is an increase in the amount of ANA, one the body's innate endocannabinoids. It also occupies proteins that transport endocannabinoids to be metabolized. The net result is an increase in endocannabinoids at CB1 and CB2 receptors.

However, CBD is a CB1 antagonist, so it tends to block effects of endocannabinoids at CB1 receptors. Because of this, we think of CBD as having primarily CB2 stimulation effects. CBD also activates other receptors that are not part of the ECS in the body's systems, that have to do with pain perception, emotions, and inflammation.

Other effects

The vast majority of marijuana's medical effects occur by impacting the ECS. However, the cannabinoids in marijuana have other beneficial therapeutic effects that don't work through the ECS. Cannabinoids are potent antioxidants, showing positive effects by counteracting the adverse effects of oxidative stress. In addition, THC has been shown to block the effects of certain enzymes. Also, as discussed above, CBD can bind to receptors on cells that are not part of the ECS.

Therapeutic Targets

The primary therapeutic target of CBD in the body and brain is to reduce inflammation. It is inflammatory processes, especially chronic inflammation, that underlies many chronic degenerative and age-related conditions. Inflammation is a healthy physiologic response to tissue injury from trauma, toxins, infection, radiation, oxidative stress, and genetic effects, but excessive inflammation can be problematic.

The initial phase of inflammation is characterized by dilated blood vessels in the area, the release of chemicals that promote inflammatory fluids that result in swelling and effusions, and the migration of white blood cells into the area that eventually die and end up as pus. This initial phase is followed by the egress of the white blood cells, reduction of inflammatory fluids, and restoration of normal physiologic functioning.

If the condition causing the inflammatory response is not resolved, the process evolves towards chronic inflammation that can last indefinitely. Chronic inflammation is an unhealthy process that results in chronic presence of inflammatory fluids and white blood cells slowly destroying the local cells and tissues. Research has shown that chronic inflammation is important in the causation of many neurodegenerative disease, cardiovascular disease, diabetes, obesity, autoimmune diseases, and cancer.[4] [37]

Traditionally, chronic inflammation has been treated by using steroid medications and non-steroidal anti-inflammatory (NSAID) medications. These medications are all associated with significant adverse effects, including gastric irritation, renal and hepatic injury, asthma and hemolytic anemias[38] [39].

Autoimmune conditions

Autoimmune diseases are due to the body's immune system, cellular and/ or inflammatory chemicals attacking healthy cells. A few examples of autoimmune disease include Multiple Sclerosis (MS), Lupus, Rheumatoid arthritis (RA), Crohn's, and Hashimoto's thyroiditis.

The current treatment for these diseases includes inflammation-reducing medications, including NSAIDs, steroids, and toxic immunosuppressive drugs. These categories of drugs, while effective, are associated with significant and sometime life-threatening adverse effects. CBD has well-documented immunosuppressive effects on white blood cell damage and inflammatory chemicals via the ECS; as such, CBD can be an adjunct to current approved treatment for autoimmune conditions and can reduce the dose or need for certain more dangerous drugs.

There are several studies in animals and humans to support the use of CBD in the treatment of psoriasis, an autoimmune disease. A topical formulation of CBD can be used once to twice daily on the affected areas for local effects. This topical CBD can be supplemented with sublingual or vaporized CBD[17 88]. CBD has been shown in an animal model of autoimmune arthritis to improve pathologic changes in joints[40]. In addition, as discussed previously, CBD has shown anti-inflammatory effects on swelling, inflammation and inflammatory pain that are similar or superior to those of many OTC drugs currently available on the market.[15]

Multiple sclerosis (MS) results from autoimmune destruction of the myelin sheaths around large nerves. A mouse model of MS treated with CBD revealed reduction in the infiltrate of immune cells to the brain parenchyma and decreased inflammatory cell activation. Moreover, CBD treatment has been shown to have a long-lasting effect; a follow-up study 80 days after treatment revealed restoration of nerve function similar to the normal mice.

Routes of administration

There are many ways to get cannabinoid medication into the body. The way that the cannabinoid makes it into the bloodstream, and from there to the brain and the rest of the body is very important. There are four primary routes of administration: inhalation, ingestion, mucous membrane absorption and topical application.

Inhalation

Inhalation implies smoking or vaporizing cannabis flower, hashish or oil. When the material is smoked, it is actually combusted, and many products of combustion go along with the vaporized oil into the lungs. Only about 20% of the smoke is actually cannabis oil; the remainder is a hodgepodge of potentially carcinogenic hydrocarbons and inert plant particulates. However, several reputable studies have failed to find an association with long-term smoking of cannabis and increased rates of respiratory tract cancer. It is believed that the anti-cancer effects of THC and CBD probably cancel out the adverse effects of the carcinogens, but this matter has not been clearly settled with high-quality studies.

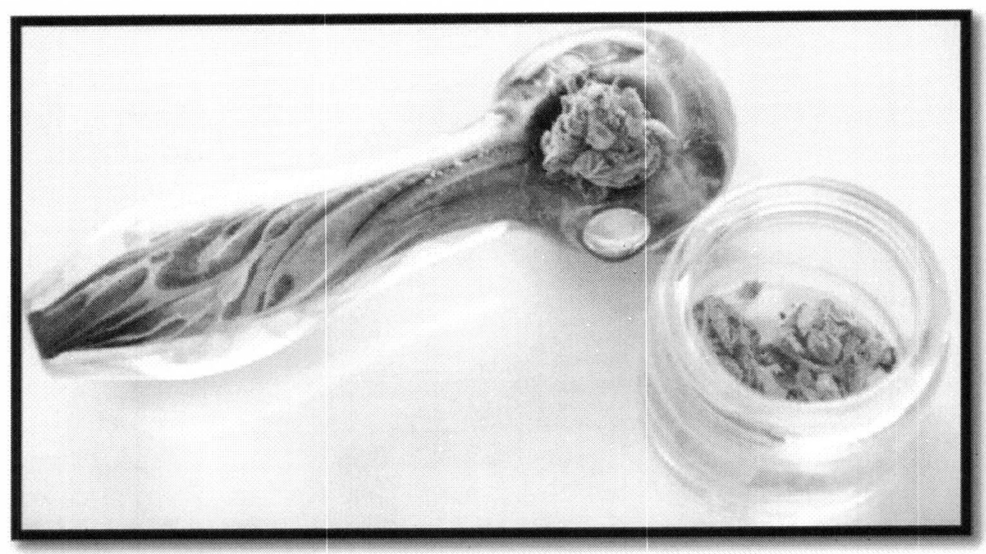

When the bud, hashish or oil is heated to a certain temperature (usually around 320-360 degrees Fahrenheit), there is no combustion, only vaporization of the cannabinoids and terpenes, along with a very small quantity of potentially carcinogenic hydrocarbons that are naturally present in the plant material.

Smoking cannabis results in incineration of half of the bud, so that only half of the oils in cannabis actually make it into the lungs. Vaporizing is much more effective, resulting in as much as 90% of these oils reaching the lungs.

Inhalation leads to direct and rapid entry into the bloodstream via the lungs, resulting in effective concentrations of cannabinoids in the bloodstream within a few minutes, and maximum effect within 15 minutes. However, beneficial effects only last 60-90 minutes. Because of its rapid entrance into the body, inhalation is good for immediate relief of pain, inflammation or spasm. An inhaled dose usually starts having effects within minutes, and usually lasts about 1-1/2 hours.

Ingestion

Ingestion implies eating, drinking or swallowing droplets of a tincture or an extract into the mouth. The medication is usually extracted with coconut or olive oil (an extract), or with alcohol (a tincture). There are also cannabis-infused drinks and cooked or baked 'edibles', or ingestible cannabis can come in the form of a tablet or capsule. The medication has to go through the stomach and into the small intestine, where it is metabolized by the liver before arriving in the bloodstream. This process is much slower, with the onset of action occurring 1 ½ -2 hours from ingestion.

This slow onset is known as the "first-pass effect", a phase that you may hear often throughout this book. It refers to the fact that when a medication is swallowed, it goes into the intestine and is passed through the liver. In the liver, the CBD and THC are metabolized to different chemicals; THC is metabolized to 11-OH-THC, and CBD to 7-OH-CBD and CBD-7-oic acid. The end result is that only about 10% of these chemicals are available after it goes through the liver; the rest are broken down into inactive metabolites due to the 'first-pass effect". In the case of THC, it is metabolized into 11-OH-THC, which is actually far more potent than regular THC.

In summary, the effects of ingested vs. inhaled cannabis medication can be quite different, as well as the length of time it takes for the CBD to start having a therapeutic effect. Ingested cannabinoids tend to work for much longer than inhaled cannabinoids, lasting up to 6 hours in the body. It is for this reason that ingested medications are particularly useful for chronic, constant pain or inflammation, or for use at bedtime to get relief all night long.

Mucous Membrane Absorption

There are several preparations of cannabinoid medications that are meant to be absorbed via a mucous membrane: the nose, the mouth cavity, or the rectum. For the nose and mouth, it is usually in the form of a spray or mist, which is inhaled through the nose or sprayed inside the mouth. For the rectum, it is usually a rectal suppository.

When cannabinoid medication is meant to be taken via mucous membrane absorption, it is usually absorbed into the bloodstream through local absorption through thin and very vascular mucous membranes, so these medications tend to be absorbed more quickly than ingested and tend to work longer than inhaled medications. They are absorbed within 30 minutes, much faster than edibles, but last 2-3 hours, shorter than an edible. However, there is no "first-pass" effect, so they are not broken down into metabolites right away as edibles are.

Extracts and tinctures can function as two different medications: Slow-release or fast-release. If the extract is placed on the tongue and then swished around the front of the mouth with the tongue, then it will absorb rapidly and miss the 'first-pass effect.' This results in rapid onset of symptom relief that lasts 1-2 hours. If the same extract is swallowed immediately, or put into a tea and ingested, then it will go through the 'first-pass effect', absorb more slowly, and last much longer.

Topical Application (Applying directly to the skin)

Cannabis-infused topicals have been used for hundreds of years and have been shown to be particularly useful for a wide array of skin conditions, fibrotic conditions just under the skin, and locally inflamed or arthritis joints.

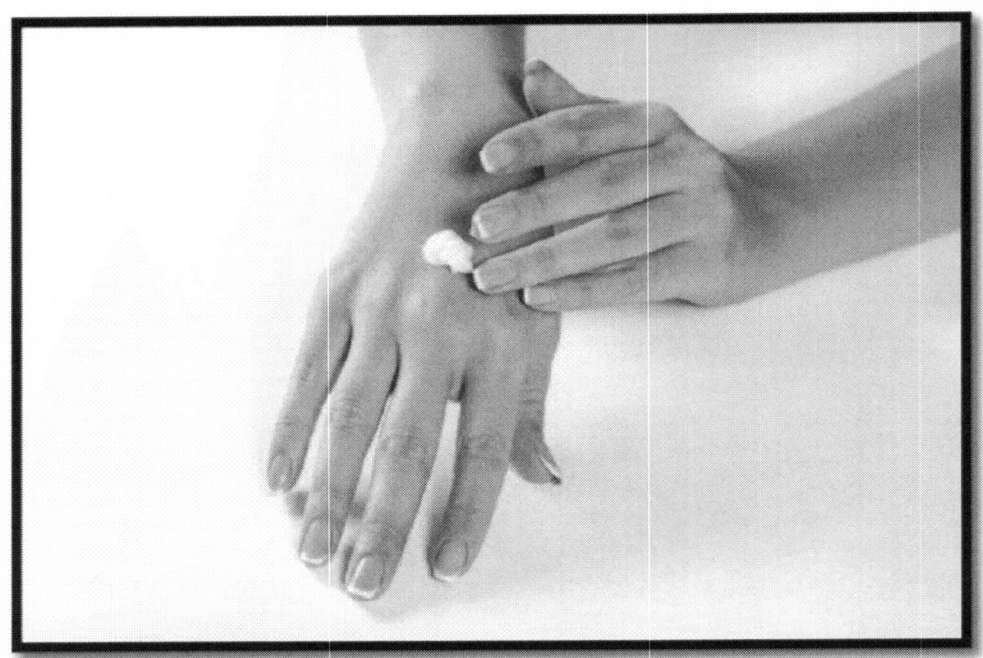

Hemp oil that is high in CBD is extracted and infused into a wide variety of vehicles, such as creams or lotions (water soluble), ointments or balms (fat soluble), sprays, lubricants, infused rubbing alcohol, or dermal patches that are applied to the skin. Because the cannabis oils are fat-soluble, they don't penetrate very deeply into the tissues, and tend to work just on the skin and the tissue just under the skin; since there is little or no absorption of the cannabis into the bloodstream with these topical preparations, there are none of the side effects, such as euphoria, anxiety, or addiction, that people sometimes worry about when using inhaled or ingested cannabis.

Topical formulations of cannabinoid medications can work in one of two ways. They are either meant to be a salve, where they are absorbed only locally by painful or inflamed tissues (for example, over a painful arthritic joint or inflamed skin conditions,) or formulated for slow release in a gel or patch form. Cannabinoid salves are often combined with other active ingredients like camphor, menthol and capsaicin, which also have local effects on pain and inflammation.

The other variety of topical cannabinoid medications, gels and patches, are meant to result in a constant slow absorption of cannabinoids through the skin and into the bloodstream. These topical cannabinoids have a very slow onset of action, and result in a constant low level of cannabinoids medication for up to 24 hours with one application. However, their absorption is highly variable from person to person.

There are plenty of CB1 and CB2 receptors in the skin, in the tissues immediately under the skin, and around the joints of the hands, feet, elbows, knees, and shoulders that can absorb CBD applied topically over a local area. Only a small amount, about the size of a dime, is needed. It should be rubbed in with deep pressure to leave a thin layer over the inflamed skin or joint.

Sources of high-quality CBD products

It is important to have a working knowledge of how the medication can be purchased online or at a store, without a prescription, in all 50 states. As was discussed previously, the CBD oil in the legal product must originate from hemp (*cannabis sativa* that is >0.3% THC), grown either outside of the US or legally within the US under the 2018 Farm Bill.

There are a myriad of websites that can be helpful for finding legal CBD, either at a nearby location, or for purchase online. Here are a few of my personal recommendations:

- www.TheHempDepot.org
- www.CBDoilreviews.com
- www.AmericanRemedyHemp.com

Flowering Bud

Smoking or vaporizing cannabis is most useful for episodic need for the medication for acute flare-ups of pain, spasms, seizures, and anxiety. Medical-grade hemp flower can generally be found in CBD stores or purchased in a dispensary in a state with medical or recreational cannabis laws. CBD extracts, tinctures, various types of edibles, and vaporizers are available in stores or online.

Even with the dozens of other dosing methods available, smoking remains very common, even for medical use. I believe that everyone should be familiar with the green 'bud' that is associated with marijuana. Over the decades, many different strains have been bred with a focus on maximizing the percentage of THC and/or CBD in the bud.

Because of the lack of euphoric effects of CBD, most strains or chemovars of *cannabis sativa* have been bred for increasingly higher levels of THC and subsequent lower levels of CBD. This has been further exacerbated by the fact that CBD tends to diminish the euphoria caused by THC

Until the recent discovery of the therapeutic effects of CBD, almost all past research has been focused on the quantity of THC being used for therapeutic effects. This trend has changed in the past decade or so, with much greater awareness of the importance of CBD, and the ratio of CBD to THC in medical cannabis formulations. Strains of hemp have since been developed with increasingly higher concentrations of CBD and very little THC.

There are literally hundreds of different strains of cannabis, with new ones being engineered continually. Some examples of high-CBD, low-THC strains are Charlotte's Web, AC/DC, and Cannatonic. Many strains are often named after the aromas given off by the terpenes in the bud, or by the color of the cannabis resin glands, called trichomes. CBD and THC are colorless, tasteless and odorless, so the smell and color of the bud has nothing to do with the potency of the bud.

The different strains of cannabis at a dispensary will often have a label stating the concentrations of THC and CBD, but clinicians and patients should be aware that these labels are notoriously inaccurate. Each new batch of bud may have markedly different potency, even if they came from the same dispensary and have the same name of strain. Stick to the therapeutic goal of starting out with a low dose, titrating slowly up to clinical effect.

Marijuana flower is usually ground in handheld grinder, which can be purchased at dispensaries for a few dollars. Grinding the bud into small particles makes it burn more evenly and smoothly. When the bud is heated up by a vaporizer or burned, the crystallized oil releases a fume or vapor of medication that is inhaled. Some devices used to burn marijuana flower include joints, hand pipes, bubblers, one-hitters, or water pipes ("bongs").

There are a myriad of glass, metal, and water pipes available. These can hold large amounts of ground cannabis flower, however, and are therefore not generally good for use for medical purposes.

There are also many designs of vaporizers for plant material, ranging in cost from around twenty to several hundred dollars. Many are designed to allow for precise control of the temperature, so the oils are aromatized at exactly the correct temperature. CBD oil boils at 160-180 degrees Celsius (320-356 Fahrenheit) and turns into a vapor, whereas THC oil boils at 157 Celsius (315 Fahrenheit). A joint, however, can reach 2000 degrees Fahrenheit, incinerating at least half of the bud before releasing any of the oils for inhalation, making vaporizers a preferred choice for accurate and efficient dosing.

For dosing on-the-go, a more practical alternative to a tabletop vaporizer is a handheld pen vaporizer, similar in size and design to an e-cigarette. Disposable cartridges are available for these portable vapes, containing exact amounts of CBD or whole plant extract; depending on the purity and concentration of the oil, generally, each inhalation of a pen vaporizer will provide 2.0 – 2.5mg of CBD.

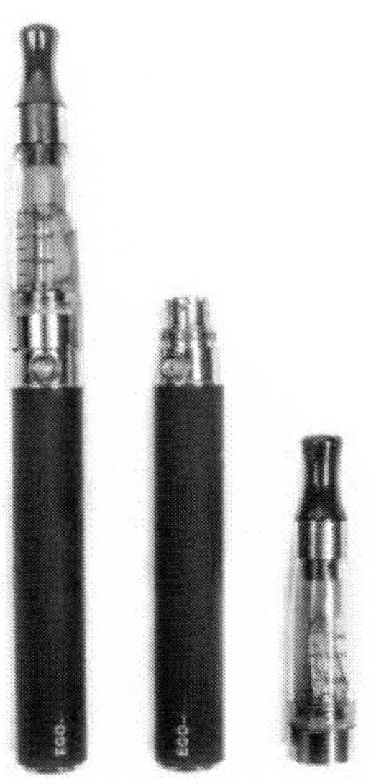

Cannabis Oil

This is a highly concentrated form of cannabinoids in the oil base made by solvent extraction. Cannabis oil usually comes in potency from 60-85 percent cannabinoids but has been reported to be as high as 99 percent cannabinoids. The oil can be consumed as an edible, but traditionally is vaporized in a specially designed device that produces the very high temperatures necessary for vaporization of the extract for inhalation. This is a much higher temperature than is required to vaporize oil in diluents.

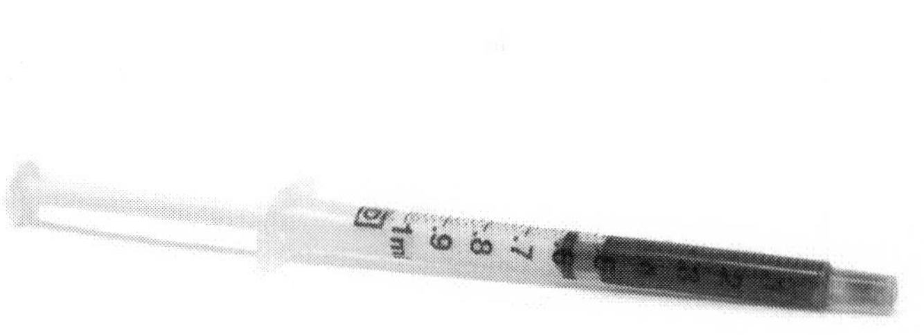

These devices vaporize CBD or whole-plant (THC and CBD) oil that has been diluted in glycerin or propylene glycol. Propylene glycol is not recommended as a diluent because of health risks when it is heated. Great care should be taken in general when sourcing these cartridges due to the prevalence of illicit or counterfeit cartridges on the market, some of which contain substances not approved for human consumption and have been shown to cause extreme adverse reactions and even death. To avoid the risk of counterfeit, these cartridges should only be purchased directly from a dispensary or reputable brand.

Cannabis oils usually contain high amounts of THC and are used for recreational purposes. This formulation is very potent and complex to administer, with huge potential of excessive euphoric effects and side effects from the THC. Therefore, it i not recommended for medication administration.

The one exception is Rick Simpson Oil, which is very high in THC, and used for 60-90 days to treat late-stage cancer.

Micro-dose Inhaler (MDI)

More recently, the CannaKit® was created with a patented micro-dose inhaler feature (MDI®). The MDI has the appearance of a cigarette or one-hitter, but it is actually a patented metal tube, the tip of which holds exactly 50mg of ground bud. This allows for precise dosing of cannabis medication, from 0.5mg to 6.0mg of inhaled medication, and dramatically reduces the amount of expensive bud that is often wasted with other means of smoking. It comes with an odor-proof carrying case, which carries a couple days' worth of ground bud, and a cleaning tool.

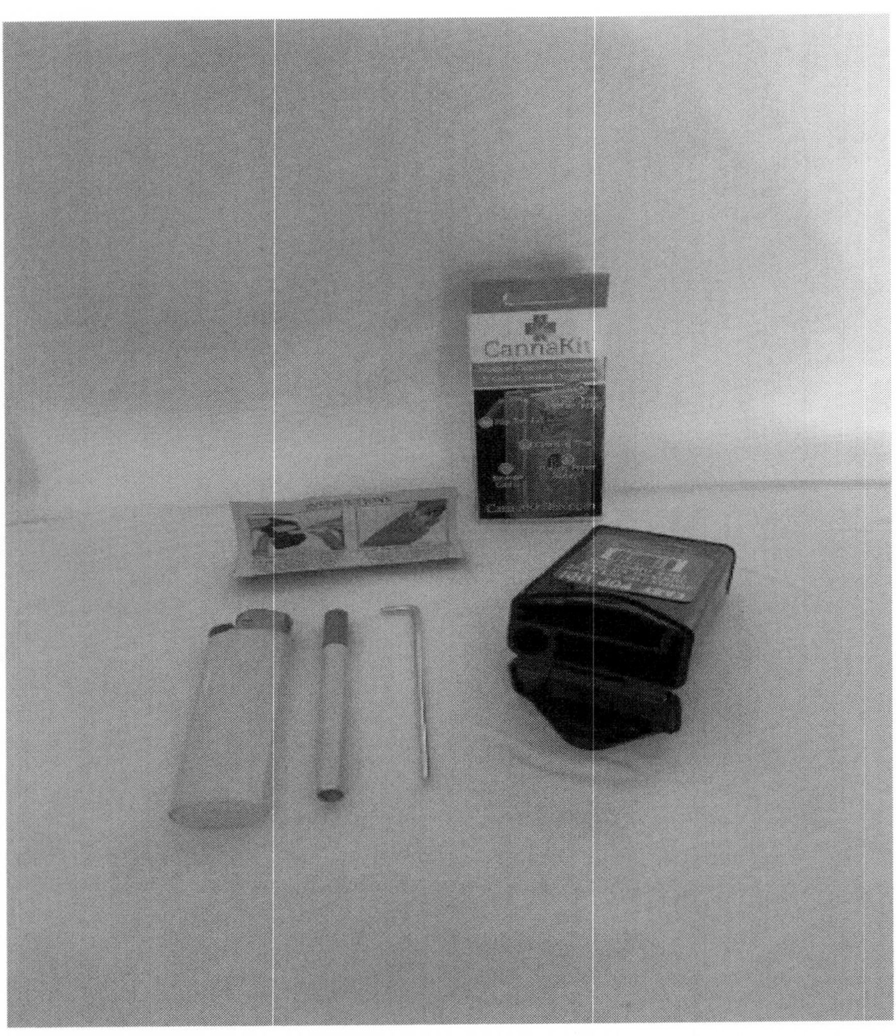

The clinical effects of cannabis medication are directly related to the amount of smoke that the patient inhales. The patient should hold the inhaled fumes in the lungs for 2-3 seconds to maximize absorption of the medication, and is advised to start with a small, deep inhalation of the fumes. When there is THC in the bud, the initial effects of the medication are usually some euphoria, setting in a couple of minutes after this initial dose.

Since CBD has no euphoric effects, there are no obvious sensations or effects initially after smoking straight CBD or hemp flower. CBD reaches a peak dose in the blood after about 9-23 minutes; it is at this time that the relaxing, anti-anxiety effects become noticeable. Because the medication is inhaled and bypasses the first-pass effect that occurs when the medication is ingested, it starts working much more quickly, but also last a much shorter duration, 1-1/2 hours.

Smoking bud for medical purposes has several pitfalls. The first is the obvious, often intense lingering aroma that is associated with the exhaled smoke. Since cannabis is still an illegal drug, even when used for medical purposes, and the fully legal, medical grade >0.3% THC hemp strains produce the same aromas as full-spectrum *cannabis sativa;* this similarity can result in legal and social issues from the use of CBD flower.

The second pitfall is that the cannabis smoke is made up of hundreds of by-products, some of which are known respiratory tract irritants, so that the clinician wouldn't want to recommend use of smoked bud in patients with certain respiratory tract conditions, or for use in and around children or people with respiratory tract conditions.

It is important to note, however, that the smoke-related by-products of smoking cannabis have not been associated with increased rates of respiratory tract cancer. Also, vaporizing the bud at lower temperatures, instead of igniting the bud when smoking it, releases much higher concentrations of the pure medicine with markedly fewer byproducts.

Hashish

Cannabis hashish, or "hash", is an opaque, waxy substance made from the compressed resin glands of the cannabis bud. Hash has been around for almost as long as humans have been smoking cannabis, and has a long history of medical use.

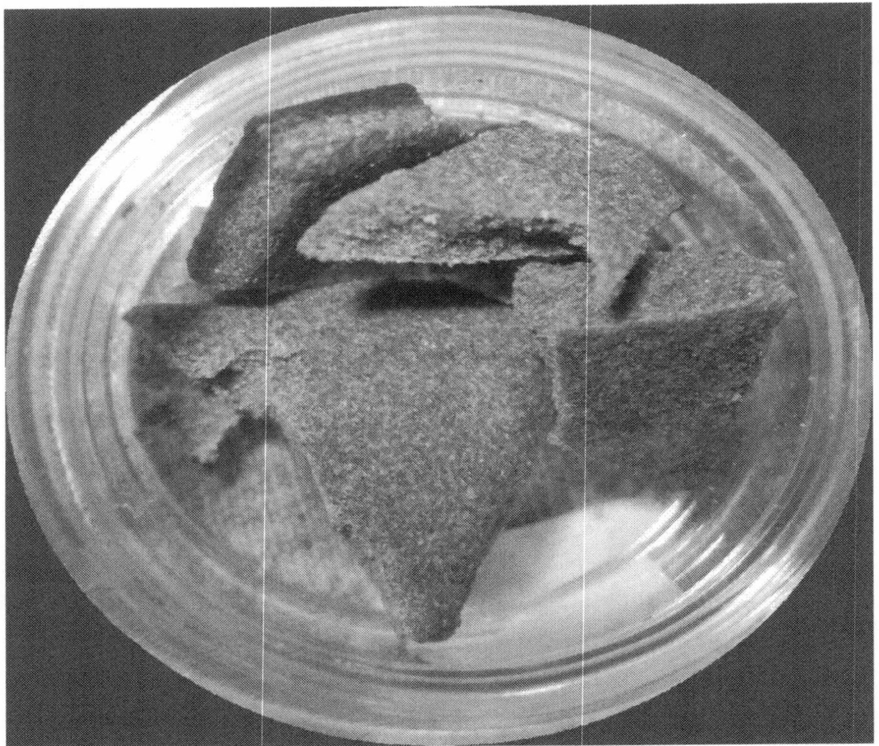

It contains all the same active ingredients as cannabis flower, but hash is far more concentrated. Like cannabis flower, hashish is traditionally smoked or vaporized. The exact hardness of the hashish varies significantly, depending on how it is prepared.

It can be hard and waxy, soft and pasty, or come as an oil. The color ranges from earthy brown to tan to yellowish red. Hashish is a much more concentrated form of cannabinoids and terpenes than the bud, so the dose needs to be adjusted so as not to get too much medication with each inhalation.

Cannabis Tinctures and Extracts

Cannabis tinctures are alcohol extractions; the other vehicles for extracting include coconut and vegetable oils. These liquids contain concentrated CBD or both THC and CBD, but also contain all of the other important organic chemicals in the plant, including other cannabinoids, terpenes and flavonoids. These liquids are often green from chlorophyll or honey-colored and may have an unpleasant taste and smell. Certain extraction techniques minimize the amounts of terpenes and chlorophylls in the tincture. Most tinctures and extracts are produced locally, and do not meet the high level of consistency and quality control that come with large-scale manufacturing organizations.

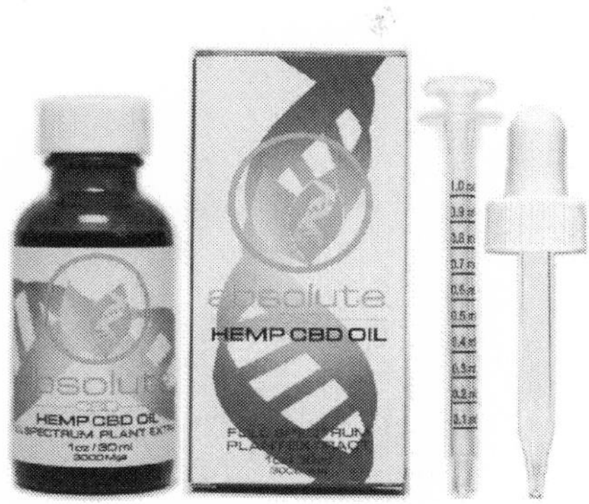

Until cannabis was banned in 1937, pharmaceutical cannabis tinctures were the second most common medication available at pharmacies. It is interesting to note that in the states where medical cannabis has been legal the longest, the trend of cannabis use has been away from smoked or vaporized cannabis, and towards its use as a tincture or edible. This could be because of the perceived negative effects from smoking and associated social issues with the aroma of smoked or vaporized medicine.

Tinctures and extracts do not work as quickly as smoked or vaporized medicine, but they have a more rapid onset of action compared to other ingested forms of the medicine. The tincture is an approximately 75% alcohol vehicle that is delivered via a dropper under the tongue, where more rapid absorption occurs via sublingual arteries. The drug misses much of the first-pass effect from the liver. Like smoked or vaporized medication, its effects come on quickly, dissipating rapidly within a few hours.

In addition, the precise measurements afforded by a dropper or oral syringe and the precise concentrations of the tincture or extract lead to consistent dosing for the patient. It is important to advise the patient not to swallow the preparation, as this will cause it to go through the GI tract to the liver and undergo the first-pass effect. If the tincture is added to a tea or liquid, then it absorbed as an "edible" form of the medication, with the slow and gradual onset of effect associated with all cannabinoids that go through the GI system.

The type of cannabinoids present (THC and/or CBD) and their concentrations should be documented on the packaging. As with cannabis flower, these labels are often incorrect if the product does not have high standards of preparation, manufacturing, and quality control.

Cannabis Butter and Edibles

Cannabis butter is a soft, light green, butter-textured substance that is made from cooking the cannabis bud with butter to extract the cannabinoids into the butter. It is often used as an ingredient to cook and bake a wide variety of cannabis edibles. In addition, there are an increasing variety of candies and flavored drinks that have extracted cannabinoids in them.

The cannabinoids are digested in the GI tract and go through the first-pass effect of the liver. This means that the time it takes to have an effect is much longer, about one to two hours, and that the effects last much longer, five to six hours. Approximately 85% of CBD is metabolized into inactive compounds by the first-pass effect, so orally ingested CBD is less effective than CBD administered via other routes.

Edibles and cannabis butter have several positive aspects: They have a slow onset of action and prolonged duration or effect, making them ideal for chronic pain control or nighttime dosing. In addition, when THC is ingested and is metabolized by the liver, it is actually converted to a different substance called 11-hydroxy-THC, which is many times more psychoactive than the delta-9-THC that comes from inhaled cannabis.

Edibles are hard to dose because of the large variation in the batches of cannabis butter produced by small operations. Also, the amount of active ingredients in the edible decreases with longer duration of exposure to stomach acids. The presence or absence of food in the stomach can likewise affect absorption and clinical effects.

Eating too many milligrams of THC, not CBD, can cause dysphoria, a highly unpleasant sensation akin to agitation, panic, or impending doom. People often go the emergency room when the dysphoria is very bad or prolonged. Like all products found in the dispensary, the amount of THC and CBD in the product may be incorrect due to problems with quality control and manufacturing in small start-up companies, so it is wise to exercise caution with edibles, especially when they are from small "mom-and-pop" manufacturers.

Once again, when dosing and titrating cannabis edibles, start with a low dose. First, eat a small piece of the edible and wait a while to let it take effect; If no substantial effect is felt, increase slowly until you feel comfortable with the correct dose for the condition. Edibles can be hard to titrate because of the slow onset of action and long duration of effect.

Another issue with edibles is that there are few standards for labeling and packaging for these products. A recent informal analysis of several popular brands of edibles in Colorado found the products sold by several manufacturers to contain significantly lower concentrations of cannabinoids than what was listed on the label. In time, new regulations and enforcement will result in higher quality and standards for edibles; for the meantime, however, the patient will have to become familiar with dosing different brands of edibles.

Edibles that contain THC have also recently come under fire for safety concerns. Because they usually come is simple packaging, and are often marketed as tasty treats, such as baked goods, candy or soft drinks, this has resulted in a spike in the number of children mistakenly ingesting the edible and ending up in the emergency room. There have yet to be any reported deaths, but serious side effects have been known to occur. Due to this concern, harsher regulations on the sale of edibles are now being enforced, mandating accurate labeling and requiring single-wrap servings to prevent accidental overdose.

CBD-only products, on the other hand, even in very high doses of hundreds of milligrams, have no appreciable side effects or euphoria. All cannabis medications should still be clearly and accurately labeled with THC and CBD content by percentage, as well as proof that the product has passed a "Safety Screen" for microbes, fungi, and pesticides. For extracts and edibles, these labels wouldn't have a percentage of THC or CBD, but the number of milligrams of CBD and THC per dose or serving.

CBD Isolates vs. Whole-Plant Extracts

The majority of CBD products available in stores or online are made with isolated CBD. This pure CBD has been extracted from hemp oil and has only tiny amounts of the other cannabinoids and terpenes in the oil. The FDA-approved medicine Epidiolex® is one of these, consisting of 99.5% pure CBD. Usually these isolates are very clear and tend to have no smell or taste, since CBD is odorless and tasteless. Epidiolex® uses sesame seed oil as the vehicle and has flavors added to it.

The preferred CBD products, however, are not isolates, but are made from whole plant extract known as broad-spectrum. These extracts range from 3-30% CBD, and the rest of the oil is non-THC cannabinoids, such as CBG, CBN, CBC, THCV, and many terpenes. These broad-spectrum extracts tend to be dark green, and often have a fruity or earthy flavors and aromas due to the presence of terpenes.

A 2015 study from Israel directly challenges one the main premises of big pharmaceutical companies who claim that artisanal botanical "whole plant" extracts are inherently inferior to pure isolates. The study, conducted by one of the scientists who discovered the components of the ECS, showed that isolates of CBD have a "bell-shaped" curve when it comes to dosing.[13] That is, as the dose of CBD goes higher, therapeutic effects tend to increase, but only to a certain point, at which the therapeutic effect plateaus; with the administration of a higher dose, the effects are actually lessened.

In the study, they used a broad-spectrum extract that was 17.9% CBD, with tiny percentages of many other cannabinoids and terpenes, compared to an isolate of CBD similar to Epidiolex®. The broad-spectrum extract had a direct dose-dependent response to pain and inflammation; that is, as the dose increased, so did the benefit, and there was no drop-off as the dose went higher. Of course, at a certain dose of CBD, there were no additional therapeutic benefits. This makes whole plant extract a preferable way to dose CBD.

The researchers also found that a lower dose of CBD was needed to get the same benefits for pain or inflammation reduction. The researchers felt that the whole plant extract was a superior medication due to the "entourage effect" of the other cannabinoids and terpenes on the ECS receptors. For this and other important reasons, only broad-spectrum (also known as whole-plant) extracts of CBD are recommended.

THC dysphoria

As mentioned before, accidentally taking an excessive dose of THC can, and does, commonly occur with recreational use of cannabis, especially with poorly manufactured edibles, resulting in a significant number of emergency room visits for THC-induced dysphoria, a very unpleasant sensation of impending doom, often associated with marked disequilibrium and ataxia. Recent evidence suggests that CBD can be used in the acute treatment of THC-induced dysphoria, as CBD acts as a potent antagonist of the actions of THC.[42] A large single dose of 200mg of CBD sublingually is recommended to resolve THC induced dysphoria.

Chapter 4:
How Safe is CBD?

In a nutshell, CBD is extremely safe. It is essentially a plant oil, not unlike sunflower or olive oil; the main difference is that CBD interacts with the ECS. CBD in particular blocks an enzyme and fills transport proteins that ends up increasing the amount of our naturally produced endocannabinoids in our body; so, at a glance, CBD is not only extremely safe, but a natural and essential component to the body's normal, healthy functioning.

Hemp Oil

CBD is legal and available in all 50 states without a prescription if it is sourced from low-THC 'hemp' plants grown under the auspices of the 2018 Farm Bill. When it is extracted from these low-THC cannabis or hemp plants, it is considered by the federal government as a nutritional supplement that is 'generally recognized as safe' (GRAS) by the FDA.

Extraction techniques

There are several extraction techniques. Often, for the 99.5% pure CBD oil, the original hemp or cannabis oil has undergone several different extraction techniques. The use of organic solvents, such as butane and propane, can leave behind a residue that is inhaled or ingested along with the CBD. It is recommended that only cold CO2 extraction methods be used, but no matter what method is used, certified laboratory analyses of the marijuana bud, extract, or tincture should be freely and readily accessible by the consumer, either online or at the dispensary.

Contaminants

Until recently, there were no federal laws and few state laws regarding testing for contamination of hemp or marijuana oil. The new 2018 Farm Bill has changed this situation, and now the FDA is responsible for ensuring that all CBD products meet appropriate safety and quality standards.

In addition to the residues of organic solvents used to extract the oil from the plant material, there are several other significant contaminants to be concerned about. These include pesticides, heavy metals, microorganisms such as mold, and aflatoxins from fungi. Repeated low-level exposure to any of these contaminants can have serious health effects. Again, any legitimate dispensary should be able to provide laboratory results that certify the absence of heavy metals, pesticides, microorganisms, and fungi.

Prior to the 2018 Farm Bill in the US, the FDA did not have oversight of CBD artisanal products, and the vast majority of CBD extracts and topicals on the market were of poor quality, due to a number of reasons, including:

- Lack of certified Good Manufacturing Practices (GMP)
- Poor consistency of potency from batch to batch
- Inadequate potency of number of milligrams of CBD for a therapeutic effect
- Contamination with fungi, pesticides, or heavy metals
- Poor or inaccurate labeling and packaging

Some of these poor-quality products are still available, and their low cost often makes them more desirable to uneducated consumers. Over time, FDA enforcement should make these inferior products obsolete.

Consistency

Most high-CBD cannabis bud or hemp and CBD products will have significant variation in the potency from batch to batch. This is because cannabis is a plant, so the amount of CBD oil that it produces will naturally vary based on different growing conditions. CBD edibles, tinctures, and other products tend to be manufactured by small companies and often have issues with product consistency from batch to batch.

For CBD-only products, this is not a concern, because if one batch is slightly weaker than another, it will soon become apparent to the person using the medication, and the dose can easily and safely adjusted. With THC, however, this is a different matter, because even small changes in doses of THC by a few milligrams can result in side effects and euphoria,

The few existing manufacturers of high-quality CBD products test each batch for consistency and contaminants when the oil is initially processed and at the end of the manufacturing process. They also send batches of their products to independent laboratories for analysis. This breakdown of chemical content is known as the Certificate of Analysis, abbreviated COA. Most legitimate companies will have a QR code on their product so that consumers can immediately see the results of the COA.

Side effects

For all intents and purposes, in the dose ranges that are discussed in this book (20mg to 200mg a day) there are few and mild side effects. There are some pleasant associated effects, such as mood elevation, anxiety/stress relief, reduced inflammatory pain and stiffness from arthritis, and overall body relaxation, but none of these impair the brain or one's ability to drive, think or operate devices, nor are they associated with cancer or any other chronic disease or addiction.

There are several large, high-quality randomized clinical trials (RCTs) using large doses of CBD over prolonged periods of time demonstrating that CBD does not have the effects of euphoria, impaired coordination, driving, operating dangerous machinery, or issues with concomitant use of alcohol.[14]

Unfortunately, Epidiolex® is only approved for use by the FDA if swallowed (ingested). Because 90+% of the CBD is metabolized by the first-pass effect into inactive metabolites when CBD is ingested, the recommended maintenance dose of Epidiolex is huge, 1600mg a day. These very large doses of CBD have been associated with liver function elevations in up to 16% of the patients who are using CBD concomitantly with potentially toxic seizures medications.

It is not clear if the liver elevations are due to the CBD itself, or to the 33 different metabolites of CBD that may be liver irritants. In any case, th liver function elevations resolve with discontinuation of Epidiolex®. It may also be that some seizure medications have drug interactions with CBD, thereby causing the liver irritation.

Recent reports suggest that 7% of the US population use CBD regularly.[15, 16] There has been no reported association of liver function elevation with low doses of CBD (20mg-200mg a day) when using CBD sublingually or by vaporizing.[17]

According to the 2017 World Health Report on CBD, "CBD is generally well tolerated with a good safety profile. Reported adverse effects may be as a result of drug-drug interactions between CBD and patients' existing medications. To date, there is no evidence of recreational use of CBD or any public health related problems associated with the use of pure CBD."[18, 19]

CBD has no effect on a wide range of physiological and biochemical parameters or significant effects on animal behavior unless extremely high doses are used. Effects on the immune system are less clear: there is evidence of immune suppression at higher concentrations, but immune stimulation may occur at lower concentrations.[18, 20]

Rare cases of low platelet levels and thrombocytopenia were reported in human studies of Epidiolex®. Both CB1 and CB2 receptors are found on platelets; however, there is currently no clinical explanation for the rare occurrence of thrombocytopenia in the Epidiolex® studies.

CBD has remarkably few, and mostly mild, adverse effects. At low doses, CBD is mildly stimulating, similar to a cup of coffee. Long-term use is associated with decreased perception of stress and anxiety, and improved overall mood. CBD does not cause addiction or dependency, nor does it create the sensation of euphoria or getting 'high.' Contrary to its recreational counterpart, THC, CBD does not carry the risk of negative side effects such as physical dependency, anxiety, agitation or psychosis.

Taking CBD with Other Medications

CBD can affect the cytochrome P450 system in the liver that has to do with metabolism of about 75% of the known FDA-approved medications. Laboratory studies have shown that CBD is a potent inhibitor of several of the enzymes that metabolize other drugs, but it is not clear if these laboratory studies are relevant to what happens in humans with therapeutic doses of CBD.

Approximately 90% of orally-ingested CBD is metabolized via the first-pass effect, resulting in dozens of CBD metabolites. The much higher doses used with oral Epidiolex® can result in pharmacologically relevant concentrations of these metabolites. There is very little research on the effects of CBD metabolites.

CBD use can increase the levels and prolong the effects of blood-thinning medications, such as warfarin. There is a case report of Epidiolex® causing a clinically significant interaction with warfarin; during initiation and titration of CBD in patients using warfarin and/or seizure medications, close blood monitoring is recommended.

Again, only in the Epidiolex® studies, dose-related elevations of liver transaminases were seen with concomitant use of the seizure medications of Valproate and Clobazam. These elevations resolved with discontinuation of Epidiolex®.

For both thrombocytopenia and elevated liver transaminases, it is important to note that these studies were unusual. The CBD isolate was administered in very high doses, up to 1600mg/day taken orally, and to subjects who were already on multiple seizure medications. These very high doses would impact the liver enzyme systems much more than the lower doses used with artisanal formulations, usually 1/20th the dose.

Like grapefruit, watercress, goldenseal, and St. John's wort, CBD can impact drug metabolism by decreasing certain liver enzyme activity, potentially increasing the plasma concentration of the prescribed drugs. This adverse effect is of most concern with certain seizure drugs and blood thinners. Your medical professional should review which medications you are taking and consider their safety and efficacy when used in combination with CBD, but remember that the vast majority of physicians and nurses have had no education about the ECS, THC or CBD.

Allergic Reactions

Just like other weed pollens, such as ragweed, marijuana pollen may be allergenic to some users. There are hundreds of byproducts in smoke that could potentially trigger an allergic reaction. In addition, people may have an allergic reaction to common contaminants of non-medical-grade cannabis flower, such as mold, fungi, or pesticides.

Although still uncommon, there is an increasing number of reports of allergic reactions to marijuana bud and marijuana-based medications. The most common allergy symptoms would be runny nose, nasal congestion, sneezing and a dry cough. Swelling/itching around the eyes and hives on the skin have also been reported. There have even been reports of severe anaphylactic allergic reaction after eating a marijuana edible, but these cases are few and far between.

Some studies have suggested that exposure to hemp pollen in large outdoor grow operations can result in people becoming allergic to marijuana pollen. If you think you are having an allergic reaction to marijuana bud or extract, discontinue use immediately and bring the matter to the attention of your medical professional.

Liver Conditions

Endocannabinoids are thought to affect the liver in several ways. First, they are associated with fat accumulation through two mechanisms: increased fat formation in the liver, and decreased fat breakdown in fat tissue. CBD has no effect on appetite stimulation, or the "munchies" which are commonly associated with THC use.

Stimulation of the CB1 receptors on the liver cells are thought to promote liver fibrosis, which is associated with the increasingly common nonalcoholic fatty liver disease (NAFLD). On the other hand, CB2 receptor stimulation, which are upregulated in chronic liver disease, are thought to be protective against liver fibrosis.

Fatty liver, fibrosis, and associated late sequelae are increasingly common, and often considered part of the metabolic syndrome. Obesity and diabetes mellitus are less common in cannabis user than among the general populace, and it has been postulated that modulation of the ECS with CBD can positively impact the continuum from excess energy storage of fat in liver cells, to fibrosis and eventually symptomatic liver disease. The ECS has also been postulated to have therapeutic effects on fatty liver via anti-inflammatory effects and modification of energy metabolism via antagonism of CB1 receptors.

CBD has also been shown to improve alcohol-induced fatty liver via anti-inflammatory and anti-fibrotic effects modulated via the CB2 receptors on liver cells.

Non-Alcoholic Fatty Liver Disease (NAFLD) is a metabolic disorder (part of the metabolic syndrome) characterized by excess fat accumulation in the liver. NAFLD is the most common liver disease in the world; about one-third of US adults have been diagnosed with the condition. Excessive fat accumulation in this area can progress to steatohepatitis, fibrosis, cirrhosis and even liver cancer.

Reduction in alcohol use, an anti-inflammatory diet, weight loss, and improvement in inflammatory and metabolic markers are the current treatment for early fatty liver and liver fibrosis. Animal studies of CBD with chronic and binge alcohol feeding have also shown promise, revealing that CBD attenuated alcohol-binge-induced injury, and improved alcohol-induced hepatic metabolic dysregulation and fatty liver by restoring changes in hepatic mRNA or protein. Thus, CBD may have therapeutic potential in the treatment of alcoholic liver diseases associated with inflammation, oxidative stress and fatty liver.

There are no good studies of CBD alone and non-alcoholic fatty liver disease (NAFLD), but a population-based case-control study of cannabis users and non-users revealed the prevalence of NAFLD was 15% lower in infrequent cannabis users and 52% lower in regular users compared to non-users of cannabis. Further research is needed to evaluate these initial findings.

Contraindications

Significant hepatic impairment, identified via blood tests, can increase the dose and plasma levels of CBD. Elevated liver enzymes would be a relative contraindication to use of CBD. Mild hepatic impairment does not require dosage adjustments.

Special Groups of People

As we have discussed, CBD is exceptionally safe, has few and mild side effects, and can have significant health benefits for a wide variety of conditions. However, there are certain groups of people who are at a greater risk of serious side effects from using CBD; the following groups are strongly advised to have a serious discussion with their medical professional prior to taking CBD or cannabis products and may need to take extra precautions.

Pregnant Women

As with many medications, there is very little existing research on CBD and THC use during pregnancy, specifically with regards to their potential effects on fetal development. It is known that the oils in marijuana are fat-soluble, and therefore cross easily from the placenta into the fetal blood supply, but it is unclear whether this has a notable impact on the embryo. The lack of research is unfortunate because THC has been shown to be particularly useful for the treatment of chronic nausea or ‘morning sickness’, which occurs in 70-80% of pregnant women.

One 1994 study examined expectant mothers in Jamaica who used a home-remedy of marijuana to treat the morning sickness. These subjects were compared to similar Jamaican mothers who didn’t use any marijuana, the control group. The study found no differences in birth weight, premature delivery or behaviors in infancy and childhood.

Three other, larger studies of British, Australian, and Dutch women similarly did not find any evidence that marijuana use during pregnancy had a discernible impact on the child, nor that it had any discernible impact on birth weight or premature delivery.

There are two other studies of children on marijuana use during gestation that are still ongoing. So far, these studies have shown a slight correlation between marijuana use in pregnant mothers and the occurrence of behavioral issues, lower IQ and psychotic symptoms later in their child's development; However, some of these effects are probably due to the significant confounding factors of tobacco and alcohol use among pregnant mothers, and are likely not the direct result of being exposed to marijuana.

More research on this topic needs to be done. As is the case with cigarettes and alcohol, the general consensus on the topic is that women should refrain from using marijuana during pregnancy or while trying to get pregnant, even for medical purposes. Because of the limited research of CBD in humans, and because it is a fat-soluble drug that crosses into the placenta and breastmilk, the use of CBD is not recommended in pregnant women, women actively trying to become pregnant, and breastfeeding mothers.[23 42]

Children

The brain continues to undergo important development up until age 25, so it is likely that marijuana use in anyone younger may have long-term impact. The ECS in the brain is involved with laying down the correct nerve tracts in the brain. Excessive doses of THC have been shown in animals to affect the normal development of several nerve systems in the brain. There is some evidence in humans that regular use of THC, especially high levels of THC throughout the day, can cause structural changes in the brain, which are associated with emotional and reasoning issues.

Most of the effects of CBD occur outside of the brain, in the body's immune system. However, CBD does cross over into the brain, and there are effects in the immune system cells in the brain from CBD. CBD has been used in high doses in high-quality randomized clinical trials for the treatment of intractable seizures in infants and toddlers. These studies of these infants do not reveal any significant side effects from CBD, but once again, more research on the topic is needed.

Elderly

The elderly population will probably benefit the most from CBD. CBD has many positive effects on several conditions that are common among the elderly, such as arthritis, dementia, and cancer. Unlike THC, which can cause many unpleasant side effects such as anxiety, agitation, short-term memory loss, balance issues, and euphoria, CBD has few, if any side effects, which makes it an excellent adjunct medication for elderly patients.

Because very elderly patients often don't metabolize medications the same way as younger adults, they are advised to start at half the recommended dose for their condition and titrate up the dose very gradually.

Alcohol

Alcohol can cause euphoria, mood disturbances, balance, and coordination issues, all of which can also occur with THC. Alcohol used in high doses over a long period of time is associated with liver fibrosis and eventually potentially fatal cirrhosis. Once again, CBD does not have these side effects. CBD has been shown to decrease the brain degeneration associated with long-term alcoholism, and to reverse liver fibrosis in certain clinical situations. Studies in mice have shown that taking CBD after binge drinking had a protective effect on the liver. It has been recommended to take 20-50mg of CBD as a preventative; however, further studies need to be conducted to solidify this evidence.

Drug Addiction and Dependencies

People with a history of drug/alcohol addiction or other forms of chemical dependency are strongly cautioned against using THC. It has been shown that up to 9% of people using high doses of THC daily on a long-term basis may develop a dependency on it. Certain factors, such as beginning THC usage during adolescence, or having a personal or family history of addiction, greatly increase the likelihood that an individual will become dependent on THC.

Fortunately, THC dependency is much less dangerous overall and easier to treat than dependency on other, harder addictive substances, such as opioids or benzodiazepines. In fact, THC "addiction" is similar in many ways to caffeine dependency, in that withdrawal from either substance may be mildly unpleasant, but it is in no way dangerous and need not be debilitating. CBD, meanwhile, is more of a neuroprotectant or supplement than it is a "drug" per se, and therefore does not carry with it the risk of addiction associated with real "drugs".

Schizophrenia or Psychosis

Repeated use of particularly high doses of THC has been associated with temporary episodes of paranoia and psychotic behavior. There is some research that shows an association between recreational THC use and the onset of schizophrenia, and therefore, persons with a family history of psychosis or a prior history of a psychotic episode are advised to not use THC.

CBD, on the other hand, has been shown to improve psychotic symptoms, and is currently being evaluated for use as a new type of antipsychotic medication. Several promising studies, in both animals and humans, have shown CBD to have significant effects on both schizophrenia and psychosis.

It is not clear exactly how CBD induces its effects, but functional MRI studies of the brain have confirmed that these effects occur in the areas of the brain associated with psychosis. In addition, the temporary psychosis caused by excessive THC can be treated with one dose of pure CBD oil, 100-200mg.

Chapter 5:
How to Use CBD

"Start low, go slow"

CBD is very safe, non-addictive, and does not cause euphoria. Its psychoactive counterpart, THC, however, comes with the potential for mild addiction, as well as problems with anxiety, agitation, coordination, and short-term memory loss. Because of all of the potential problems from THC, any use of medical marijuana containing THC of 0.3% or greater needs to "start low", beginning at a low dose, and "go slow", moving up the dose incrementally until the desired medical effect is achieved.

This dosing method does not apply to CBD-only medications. In general, there will be a recommended dose range for CBD, and you can start with this dose and increase as necessary based on the response. Try the lowest recommended dose for 4-5 days, then judge the effects before deciding to increase or titrate up by 5-10mg a day. CBD is incredibly safe, exhibiting few mild side effects well into the 100mg dose range; however, for most of the conditions that I will be discussing later on in this book, the optimum dose for effective treatment will be 100mg a day or less.

Finding the "Sweet spot"

When it comes to using THC or CBD for medical purposes, less is more. Most of the therapeutic effects from THC and CBD occur in ranges of a few milligrams. If you take too much, the excess amounts of THC and CBD in the bloodstream will literally flood the cannabinoid receptors (CB1 and CB2.) These receptors are not flooded naturally, so when this occurs, the receptors tend to sink inside the cell, leaving fewer receptors; this is known as down-regulation, resulting in more milligrams being necessary to get the same effect. This is where the concept of drug tolerance comes from. When tolerance develops, a higher dose becomes necessary to achieve the same effect, hence the adage: "less is more."

The goal to keep in mind while dosing THC or CBD is to get to the "sweet spot" or the blood level that is high enough to have a therapeutic effect, but not so high that it floods the receptors and leads to tolerance. The recommended doses of CBD in this book are designed to reach these "sweet spot" levels in an average adult; However, it is also expected that most people will still need to gradually titrate up from the initial or starting dose before they will reach their "sweet spot."

Reevaluate

After starting a dosing regimen of either THC or CBD, it is necessary to re-evaluate the condition to see if the dose of medication is having its desired effect; if not, upping the dose slightly is recommended. Unlike other medications, like aspirin or blood pressure regulators, THC and CBD do not cause a measurable effect immediately.

It may take several days to get to the dose with measurable effects. Generally, it is good to re-evaluate after 4-5 days if the dose is working. Once you get to the dose that is working for you, then you can begin to re-evaluate less frequently, such as every 3-6 months.

A diary is a good way to track the progress of your dose or medication. Document the dose taken, how it is taken, the time of day, and any changes in symptoms you may have experienced. After 4-5 days, you can look at the diary to get an idea of how the dose is working for you, and you can make adjustments accordingly. There are several free or inexpensive smartphone apps available to help track ones' medical marijuana use and symptom management.

Tips on Dosing CBD

Dosing CBD is probably the most challenging concept when considering therapeutic effects. In this training, we are discussing CBD extracts and topicals containing minimal or no THC. The use of CBD-only therapy is often recommended, even when THC formulations are readily available.

THC essentially has almost all the adverse effects and contraindications, such as paranoia, agitation, panic, memory issues, euphoria, and association with hyperemesis, dependency syndromes and psychosis. Therefore, many patients will prefer to see if a trial of CBD only will work.

Any medication containing THC will need to be obtained by seeing a physician certified in the state to recommend medical cannabis. Unlike CBD products, which are available in all 50 states and online, THC products cannot cross state lines and can only be obtained from dispensaries in those states that have legal cannabis.

CBD indirectly leads to an increase in quantity of the endocannabinoids by inhibiting the enzyme and transport protein that metabolize endocannabinoids. Because CBD increases the amount of naturally occurring endocannabinoid, we can think of CBD as raising the cannabinoid tone in the brain and body. The challenge here is to affect the cannabinoid tone in whichever system of the body that we are trying to treat.

The type of product you use will impact dosing requirements. CBD isolates, for instance, have a narrower therapeutic window than broad-spectrum products that contain the 'entourage' of terpenes and minor cannabinoids. As discussed earlier, CBD isolates exhibit a bell-shaped dose-response curve when administered with a narrow therapeutic window with no beneficial effect at either lower or higher doses.

Broad-spectrum CBD formulations, on the other hand, tend to show a direct correlation between dose and response, with increased doses resulting in increased responses until a therapeutic plateau is reached. Once a plateau has been reached, increasing the dose will not significantly impact the therapeutic response one way or another.

Starting Doses of CBD

When it comes to CBD, there is no one-size-fits-all dosing, as there often is with FDA-approved monomolecule drugs such as antibiotics, aspirin and NSAIDs. The starting dose of CBD should be below that dose which is expected to eventually be necessary; a good starting dose is around 10mg once a day.

This starting dose is expected to be subtherapeutic-- that is, it is not expected to result in immediate improvement of symptoms, but it is a good starting point from which to titrate up until the desired effect is achieved. The dose is increased every 4-5 days by 5mg to 10mg a day, using the detailed guidance below.

As mentioned previously, CBD has a very long half-life, approximately 1-2 days. The only reason it should be dosed more than once a day is to achieve higher plasma concentrations. For example, a dose of CBD taken orally is expected to have a low peak plasma concentration, but will last 6+ hours, while the same dose of CBD taken sublingually (under the tongue) will have a peak plasma concentration several times that of the oral dose but lasting only a couple of hours. Therefore, the number of times a day that the CBD should be dosed taken will depend on the condition and if higher peak plasma concentrations are necessary.

If the dose is not high enough, there will often be no measurable effect. The therapeutic effects will then increase as the dose increases, before reaching a "sweet spot", where maximum therapeutic benefit is achieved. As was discussed above, raising the dose above the 'sweet spot' either does nothing, or can cause the effect to drop off, resulting in fewer beneficial effects. This is because the cannabinoid receptors will down-regulate if they are flooded or overstimulated by high levels of CBD. Remember, with therapeutic effects of CBD and THC, "less is more."

When a dose of CBD gets into the bloodstream, it floods the ECS in the brain and body for several hours. The CBD is not metabolized immediately like endocannabinoids are; In fact, CBD reduces metabolism of the endocannabinoids, raising their levels. If there is constant high level of stimulation of the ECS receptors, they will down-regulate, resulting in tolerance and decreased efficacy. The goal is, therefore, to gradually titrate the dose up to the "sweet spot" where maximum effect is reached before tolerance or downregulation develops.

If the dose of CBD results in good symptom improvement, but the once-daily dose provides only a limited duration of effect, then increase the dosing to twice, then three times a day. If the duration of effect is acceptable, but the patient feels he could get further benefits from CBD, then increase the once a day dose, to get higher peak levels of CBD.

If the patient gets "breakthrough" or severe symptoms, then use a vaporized dose of CBD for rapid relief. CBD reaches peak plasma concentrations in 10 minutes. Each inhalation from a vaporizer is generally 2-2.5mg of CBD. The patient should take repeated doses after 10 minutes if there is not sufficient symptom relief.

Dosing of topical preparations for local effects can usually be done once a day because of the long half-life, and efficacy is not based on plasma levels. For long-term relief overnight, oral doses (6+ hours) can be considered. Remember, the oral dose will go through the first-pass effect, and 90% of the CBD will be metabolized to inactive metabolites, so a much larger dose may be necessary when given orally.

A few companies are now making suppositories (both vaginal and rectal) for specific conditions. Although there is little research behind using suppositories, there are plenty of persons who report benefit for menstrual cramping with vaginal CBD suppositories, and relief from inflammatory bowel diseases such as Crohn's disease using rectal suppositories. The suppositories miss the "first-pass" effect, and therefore probably deliver more medication directly to the source of the problem.

Dosing Summary

Although there are many ways to take CBD, the most recommended way is to use a broad-spectrum product. Use a vaporizer of CBD for quick onset of action (10 minutes) and short duration of effect (60-90 minutes.) Use CBD extract sublingually (under the tongue) for slower onset (30-45 minutes) but longer term effect (3-4 hours.) Only ingest CBD if other methods of using CBD aren't working. This will usually require a much higher amount of CBD.

Before starting treatment with CBD, start using a 'symptom diary'. There are several apps for your smartphone available to track how symptoms respond to medication. Find one that works for you and start tracking the most important symptoms for a couple days, before you start the CBD. Based on what you have read about CBD's effects on symptoms, identify a handful of specific symptoms that you would like to see improved with the CBD. In addition to specific symptoms such as "sharp pain," or "stiff joints," you may also want to track your general 'mood.'

Each diagnosis in this book has a recommended 'Dosing' section. Unless there are reasons to start at a different dose, start at the recommended dose. Use the diary app to track how your symptoms respond over time to this initial dose. After four days at a specific dose, you will need to determine if you should increase the dose of stay at the current dose.

If you feel that you have had maximum benefit from the CBD dose, then just continue to take this dose on a long-term basis. It is sometimes advisable to eventually taper off CBD. Many of the conditions that CBD treats might quiet down, or resolve, so that CBD is no longer necessary. If you are tapering of long-term use of CBD, it would be advisable to cut the dose in half every 4-5 days, until you get back to the starting dose, then quit.

Working with a Medical Professional

I have mentioned several times that your healthcare provider may have no knowledge or experience with using medical marijuana or CBD. If you can't convince your medical professional to help you add medical marijuana or CBD to your treatment, then you can find a compassionate, educated and experienced medical professional in your area at one of the following websites:

- www.MedicalMarijuana411.com
- www.Leafly.com
- www.MarijuanaDoctors.com
- www.AmericanRemedyHemp.com

The doctors listed at these websites have met certain criteria to be specialized in the use of THC and CBD. Make certain that they are willing to communicate with your primary care doctor so that your care and medication use is monitored correctly.

Where to get CBD Medication

Just as important as what sort of medication you are using to treat your condition, it is important to consider from whom you are getting your medication. Any medical marijuana products that contain THC will have to come from an approved dispensary. The staff at the dispensary will be able to help you find the right type of medication for your specific needs.

In general, you will be able to buy one month's worth of medical marijuana products at a time. Each month, when you go back to the dispensary, you can discuss how cannabis medication that they have recommended is working for you, and consider any adjustments that may need to be made.

The following three websites contain updated lists of all state-approved dispensaries in your area:

- www.Leafly.com
- www.MarijuanaDoctors.com
- www.WeedMaps.com

CBD is often bought online, as it is legal in all 50 states and available to be shipped across state lines. The most important consideration when shopping for CBD products is to make sure you are purchasing a high quality, contaminant-free product. There are dozens of websites offering a wide range of CBD products, but the vast majority are selling overpriced, isolate-based products that are inferior to more reliable, medical-grade formulations.

For several years now, I have been asked by patients and doctors to recommend a reliable brand of CBD products. Because of the issues discussed above, I have been very hesitant to give such recommendations in the past; however, I have evaluated many companies' manufacturing processes, laboratory testing, and relative product quality, and I now feel comfortable and confident recommending the following three manufacturers. Their products can be found for sale in retail stores around the world and online.

- www.TreevanaWellness.com
- www.TheHempDepot.com

- www.AmericanRemedyHemp.com

CBD Use and Drug Testing

A common concern among potential users of CBD products is whether their use of CBD will result in a positive result on a THC drug test; the answer to this question is a straightforward and emphatic 'no.' Drug tests that are conducted on hair and urine samples are very compound-specific, meaning that they are testing for the presence of THC and metabolites of THC, rather than the full spectrum of cannabinoids found in whole-leaf marijuana. CBD is an entirely different chemical from THC, and therefore will not show up on a drug test if one has been using CBD-only or pure hemp products.

The consumer's biggest concern in this area ought to be about the risk of buying an incorrectly labeled CBD product that is supposed to contain less than 0.3% THC, when, in fact, the actual THC concentration is much higher. Using a product that is incorrectly labeled in such a way can, and has, resulted in the user testing positive for THC on a drug test. This is yet another reason why any and all CBD products should be purchased only from well-known, high-quality manufacturers who are committed to in-depth analysis testing and accurate product labeling.

PART II: PHYSICAL DISORDERS

Chapter 6:
Chronic Pain

Chronic pain is defined by doctors as "any pain that lasts more than three months or longer than the expected tissue healing time." It is, unfortunately, a rather common condition, with more than 3 million cases reported in the US per year. While chronic pain begins without a specific cause in some individuals, many others experience it after an injury or as a side effect of another health condition, such as arthritis, back injury, migraines, or various infections. Chronic pain can originate in the brain, nerves, muscles, or at a site of trauma. The symptoms and duration of pain vary among patients, depending on individual cause and origin, and can range from acute to chronic, and mild to severe.

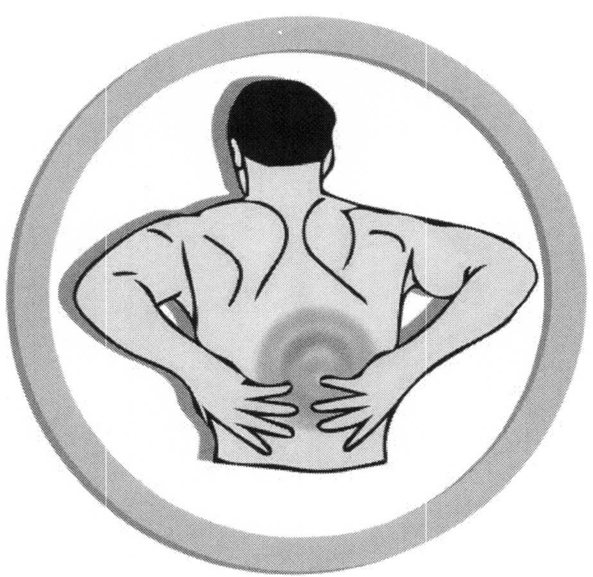

Mental health is often negatively affected by chronic pain, because living in a state of chronic pain can take a heavy emotional toll on one's daily life.

Feelings of anger, depression, low self-esteem, anxiety, and frustration can all be exacerbated by chronic pain. Because the brain processes physical and emotional pain in the same way, the depression caused by chronic pain can make the pain feel worse, which in turn reinforces the depression, thus creating a vicious cycle.

Many patients with prolonged pain end up being prescribe addictive opioid medications, such as Vicodin®, Lortab®, Norco®, Oxycontin®, Dilaudid®, and many others. The patient often ends up with both chronic pain and a severe addiction to opioids, such that they perceive worsening of pain when the opioids are withdrawn, not to mention an intense opioid withdrawal syndrome. In addition, long-term use of opioids often results in depression, insomnia, and anxiety.

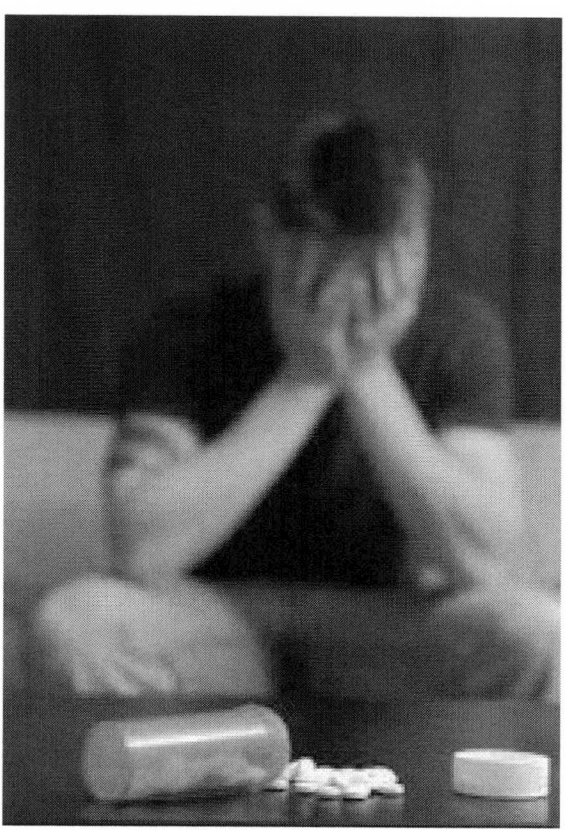

While there is no cure for chronic pain, there are a variety of treatments, ranging from medication to acupuncture and lifestyle changes, that can help alleviate symptoms so that the condition is less likely to interfere with one's daily life.

Cannabis for Chronic Pain

Medical cannabis almost always contains both THC and CBD; usually, the THC is in much higher concentrations than CBD. Unfortunately, most of the existing studies on cannabinoids and chronic pain have only looked at the benefits of combined THC, with or with or without CBD. In almost all the available studies, the dose of CBD is not provided.

THC works on the CB1 receptors in the brain and reduced perceived pain centrally from afferent spinal cord pain messaging. CBD either has no activity at the CB1 receptors or is a weak neutral antagonist of CB1 receptors. CBD is postulated to positively impact pain by decreasing inflammation and swelling via CB2 receptors, by stimulating TRPV1 receptors, and by decreasing the emotional response to chronic pain via non-ECS receptors.

There is research to support the use of CBD for all types of chronic pain, including neuropathic, centrally mediated, sympathetically mediated, and chronic persistent pain from surgery, injury, arthritis and degenerative disk conditions. The American Academy of Neurology "Guidelines" reviewed the available literature and, "based on the highest quality evidence" considering "safety and effectiveness," determined that CBD alone can help lessen centrally-mediated pain.[21]

Centrally-mediated pain includes several forms of paresthesia, burning and numbness. Also, fibromyalgia is at least partially a centrally-mediated pain condition; however, there is no clear specific pathophysiological therapeutic target in patients with this condition.

Neuropathic pain is becoming increasingly common as sequelae of HIV, Type II Diabetes, MS, and other conditions, but there still exist only a few pharmaceutical choices for the treatment neuropathic pain. Two research trials of neuropathic pain in HIV patients showed that inhaled cannabis decreased pain by 30% compared to placebo.[22] A study of intractable neuropathic pain in patients with MS, brachial plexus injury, limb amputation, and spinal cord injury found that CBD was superior to a placebo, without side effects.[23]

A study of the topical use of CBD for an animal model of arthritis confirmed that transdermal CBD gel significantly reduced joint swelling, limb posture scores as a rating of spontaneous pain, immune cell infiltration and thickening of the synovial membrane in a dose-dependent manner.[24] Evidence of tenderness returned to near baseline. Analysis of spinal cord revealed dose-dependent reductions of inflammatory biomarkers. Acute, transient joint inflammation was reduced by local CBD treatment. Prophylactic CBD treatment prevented the later development of pain and nerve damage in the arthritic joints.

As pain becomes chronic, the emotional aspects and responses to the perceived pain often become more important than the physical pain. Therefore, cognitive behavioral therapy (CBT), psychotherapy, yoga, mindfulness and relaxation techniques, as well as use of antidepressants, anxiolytics, and other therapies, can become very important as pain transitions from the subacute to the chronic phase. CBD, with 1:1 or higher ratios of CBD to THC, has been shown to positively impact mood and anxiety in patients with chronic pain.[25]

FDA-approved pain medications include non-steroidal anti-inflammatory medications (NSAIDs), short and long-acting opioids, anti-epileptic drugs (AEDs), acetaminophen (often in combination with opioids), and topical analgesics and counterirritants. Most of these medications are associated with frequent and severe adverse effects, and poor clinical support exists for their long-term use to control chronic pain conditions. Opioids in particular have serious and often life-threatening adverse effects, especially when combined with alcohol or other central nervous system (CNS) depressants, such as benzodiazepines.

Types of Pain

There are several distinct categories of pain, the determination of which can be helpful in determining the best treatment. Pain that originates at a site of injury, such as an ankle sprain or lower back strain, for example, is due to inflammation and swelling at the site of the injury. This causes achy, stiff, sore-type pain, and can often be treated best with topical pain creams or gels.

Over-the-counter topical analgesic creams can include a combination of Capsaicin, Menthol, Camphor, Lidocaine, and Salicylates.

These creams, when applied directly to the injured area, work by blocking the sensation of pain while the injured tissue is healing. If the injured area continues to be swollen, tender or stiff for more than two weeks, than a topical version of CBD cream can be used. This stimulates the CB2 receptors to block release of the chemical messengers that are causing the inflammation and swelling.

If the area of injury is particularly large or spread out, topical creams may not be useful, and an oral dose of CBD may present a better alternative. CBD is helpful in these cases because it works to decrease inflammation and swelling throughout the body, not just in a specific area. There are also beneficial anti-anxiety or mood-enhancing effects from oral CBD.

Another notable type of chronic pain is neuropathic pain. When a nerve is irritated, pinched, or injured, the nerve is damaged, which results in burning, sharp, shocking, tingling, radiating nerve pain messages, called neuropathy. These neuropathic pain messages are sent from the site of injury up to the brain, where they are perceived as pain. This is particularly common with diabetics and people with herniated disks in the neck or back.

When neuropathic pain becomes chronic, therapeutic CBD should be tried. CBD can be used topically for a small area of pain, such as the soles of the feet, or taken orally for effects in the brain, where it can reduce the pain messages coming up the spinal cord to the brain. This reduces the brain's perception of pain, similar to the way opioids work. Other nutraceuticals, discussed below, are also very helpful for neuropathic pain.

Centrally mediated pain is dysfunctional pain that develops months after a painful injury or condition. Centrally mediated pain is similar to neuropathic pain, with burning, sharp, or tingling pain, often accompanied by intolerable bursts of intense pain. This type of pain is common among sufferers of MS, Parkinson's disease, and brain or spinal cord injuries. It results in the perception of moderate to severe pain, even after an injury has healed, without any underlying physical cause; most patients who get started on long-term opioids have this type of pain.

This pain does not respond well to opioids or most FDA-approved pain medications, but there are several medicines used for depression or epilepsy that have been shown to be useful for controlling this type of pain. Unlike THC, CBD does not directly stimulate the CB1 receptors in the brain that have to do with pain perception; however, like many antidepressant medications, CBD directly stimulates serotonin receptors, resulting in an antidepressant effect. It is through this same mechanism that SSRI antidepressants such as Cymbalta®, Celexa®, Zoloft®, or another class of antidepressants known as tricyclics, such as Amitriptyline® and Imipramine®, have been shown to improve centrally mediated pain.

Fibromyalgia

Fibromyalgia is a common cause of debilitating chronic pain, often associated with insomnia and depression. It is a form of centrally mediated pain, and several researchers have suggested that fibromyalgia may be due to a deficiency in the amount of naturally occurring cannabinoids in our brain. Diminished or deficient endocannabinoid levels lead to a greatly increased perception of pain, such that even small pressure on a muscle will be perceived as painful in the brain. Likewise, decreased levels of naturally occurring endocannabinoids can result in insomnia, anxiety, and depression. The goal of treating fibromyalgia, then, is to increase the cannabinoid tone in the brain. There is more detailed discussion on ways to improve cannabinoid tone to treat this condition later on in the chapter on Fibromyalgia.

CBD Treatment

CBD has been shown to be effective in managing symptoms of chronic pain via a couple of different mechanisms. It is thought that CBD interacts with receptors in the immune system and brain, tiny proteins attached to cells that receive and aid in responding to chemical signals from different stimuli. When CBD interacts with these receptors, it creates a pain-relieving and anti-inflammatory effect, similar to that of steroid dose packs, Aleve® and Ibuprofen®. Often, chronic pain of the back or joints is caused by inflammation, and since CBD helps to reduce inflammation, chronic pain sufferers have found it to be an effective form of pain relief.

CBD also works by modifying the perception of the pain in the brain, such that the same level of pain is perceived as being lower, similar to how opioids work. Dr. Ethan Russo, a prominent CBD researcher, did a study that showed cannabinoids to be ten times more potent than morphine in a wide range of neuron-mediated pain conditions.

Finally, CBD improves how well the opioids relieve pain, so that taking CBD in conjunction with opioid medications can result in the need for approximately 30% less opioid medication to achieve the same result.

For treating localized pain, inflammation, and swelling, CBD topicals have proved to be effective. Topicals come in lotions, oils, or bath salts; some are infused with other plant extracts such as menthol, creating cooling effects. Oils are good for specific stiff spots, and bath salts relax and reduce whole-body inflammation while soaking in the tub.

When the pain is in more than just one or two specific places, CBD needs to be taken into the body via inhalation, mucosal membrane absorption of a spray or tincture, or ingestion of extracts, gummies or edibles.

Other Pain Medications that Work with the ECS

Acetaminophen (Paracetamol), which is sold by the name Tylenol®, is the most commonly used over-the-counter pain reliever. It is included in most opioid pills, such as Vicodin®, Lortab®, Norco® and Oxycodone®. Usually, 325mg of acetaminophen is added to each opioid pill for the synergistic effects, because it greatly increases the pain-relieving effects of the opioids.

Acetaminophen has been around for 100 years, but only in the past decade was it discovered how exactly it relieves pain. Once the acetaminophen enters the body, it is metabolized by the liver into a drug called AM404. The AM404 blocks the uptake of the naturally occurring cannabinoid, anandamide (ANA), resulting in increased CB1 activation by the increased levels of endocannabinoids, which, in turn, lessens the perception of pain in the brain, similar to the function of opioids. Because of this effect, acetaminophen can be used with CBD to have a separate effect on pain perception. CBD mostly decreases pain by decreasing swelling, inflammation and pain generation at the site of injury, whereas acetaminophen reduces the perception of pain in the brain.

Palmitolethanolamide (PEA) is a naturally occurring chemical in our bodies that works with the ECS and has been shown to be particularly effective of reducing neuropathic pain. Because it uses the ECS to work, it is considered a cannabinoid medication, but is not found in *cannabis sativa*. PEA works differently than CBD; it stimulates receptors inside of the cells, resulting in decreased swelling, inflammation and local pain generation at the site of injury. PEA is safe and is available as a nutritional supplement over-the-counter, usually in 400mg capsules or bulk powder.

Dosing

In general, CBD is not recommended for acute or new-onset pain. There are plenty of excellent, safe, over-the-counter oral and topical medications for treating muscle strains, sprains, bruising, and spasm. If the condition persists longer than would be expected, then CBD can be tried. Topical CBD preparations are very effective for localized painful joints and muscles. If the pain is not localized, then CBD extract swished under the tongue is beneficial. The starting dose is 10mg, three times a day. This can be doubled every 4-5 days until maximum benefit is reached. Most painful conditions don't require doses above 200mg a day.

Remember that if something continues to be painful in the body, usually there is an injury there, causing painful swelling and inflammation, and sending pain messages to the brain. So, it is not enough to just quiet the chronic pain, but the underlying cause of the persistent pain needs to be addressed. This is best done under the purview of your primary care provider.

The WebMD page on Pain Management has excellent advice and education about the possible causes of different types of chronic pain. The dosing recommendations below also include advice on how to use PEA and acetaminophen.

The following dosing advice is only for adults who are not also using any other pain medications or opioids. For advice on controlling chronic pain while using opioids, refer to the chapter on tapering off opioids with CBD.

Doses for Chronic Muscle or Joint Pain/Inflammation

Topical CBD balm: Combine equal parts CBD balm with an over-the-counter balm containing camphor, capsaicin, menthol and salicylic acid. Apply a thin layer to the affected area using very firm pressure, in the morning, afternoon, and at bedtime. Deeply massage any knots or especially tender points. Wash hands well after each application, because the capsaicin can burn mucous membranes if left on too long. Do not apply near eyes, mouth or anus. Always read the directions with the packaging for specific instructions. Topicals can be used in combination with oral medication.

Doses for centrally-mediated pain or neuropathic pain in the extremities or localized area

Topical CBD balm: Combine equal parts of topical CBD balm with an over-the-counter balm containing camphor, capsaicin, menthol and salicylic acid. Apply a thin layer to the affected area using very firm pressure, in the morning, afternoon, and at bedtime. Deeply massage any knots or especially tender points. Wash hands well after each application, because the capsaicin can burn mucous membranes if left on too long. Do not apply near eyes, mouth or anus. Always read the directions with the packaging for specific instructions. Topicals can be used in combination with oral medication. PEA and acetaminophen can be taken at same times as CBD extract.

PEA Capsules: Starting adult dose (not recommended in children:) one 400mg capsule once a day. May increase after four days to 400mg twice a day, then up to three times a day, depending on response to the medication. Once maximum pain relief has been achieved with a certain dose, maintain that dose. Maximum daily dose 1400mg.

Acetaminophen: Starting adult dose (not recommended in children:) one 625mg extended-release capsule three times a day. Prolonged or excessive use of acetaminophen can cause liver damage and other conditions. This is especially true when using acetaminophen and alcoholic beverages. Always read the package insert and consult your physician if there is any question about the appropriate use of acetaminophen. Be careful to make certain that you are not getting acetaminophen (Tylenol®) in any other medications that you are taking. The extended release versions of Tylenol® is called "arthritis pain formula", lasting eight hours and providing a more consistent control of chronic pain. This is the only dose recommended without consulting a physician. The maximum dose for acetaminophen is 3,000mg a day.

Doses for Fibromyalgia

CBD Extract: Starting adult dose (not recommended in children): 10mg of CBD extract under the tongue, in the morning, afternoon, and at bedtime. This dose may be increased by 10mg every 4-5 days depending on response to the medication. Once maximum pain relief has been achieved with a certain dose, maintain that dose. Maximum daily dose of CBD extract is 200mg.

Treatment doesn't always work

Medicine is an art, more than it is a science. Sometimes the recommended treatment doesn't work. It may not work because the combination of medications wasn't correct, or it may not work because the underlying condition causing the pain is more severe than originally thought. In these cases it is important to be patient and willing to experiment with different products and doses until pain relief is achieved.

Start out with just CBD topicals and/or extract; if after 2 weeks you are not getting enough pain relief, add the acetaminophen. Give the acetaminophen at least a week to improve the pain. Finally add the PEA capsules. If the maximum doses of these three medications are not getting you enough pain relief, it is time to go back to your physician for some advice.

Involving Medical Professionals

In most cases of chronic pain, the original cause of pain, whether it be a fracture, back strain, burn, etc. has already healed, but the pain and inflammation lingers. So the pain and the functional effects of the pain are the primary problem and the primary target of treatment. As is usually the case, most physicians will have very little knowledge of CBD, PEA or medical marijuana, and their use in chronic pain.

However, it is important to give your doctor the opportunity to assist you in finding solutions to control your chronic pain. Do not attempt to suddenly decrease or discontinue your prescription medications without consulting your doctor first. Involve your doctor throughout the process and ask her to help you gently taper off the prescription medications while you gradually titrate the dose of CBD and other medications discussed above.

Chapter 7: Headaches and Migraines

Headaches are a major public health concern with enormous individual and societal costs. Each year, about half of the population experiences headaches, including migraines (10%), tension-type headaches (38%), and chronic daily headaches (3%). With more than 3 million reported cases per year, migraines are very common in the US. Women are 1.25 times more likely to experience tension-type headaches, and 2-3 times more likely to experience migraines than men. and they tend to peak during a person's 30's.[26, 27] A migraine is a specific type of vascular headache of varying intensity that is often accompanied by nausea, vomiting, and sensitivity to light and sound. The pain caused by migraines isn't usually caused by another disorder or disease, but is believed to be due to overactivation of the trigeminovascular nervous system, which provides sensation to the face and head. Regular headaches, on the other hand, are considered to be due to muscle tension, and present entirely differently from migraines.

Migraines affect people differently, with some experiencing throbbing pain on just the right or left side of the head, while others experience pain all around the head. The pain can range from moderate to severe, but almost always interferes with daily activity. Migraine pain can last for just a few hours, or in some cases, multiple days.

While there isn't an exact cause of migraines, researchers and doctors do have some understanding of what may trigger them. Some potential triggers include hormonal changes in women, stress, drinks such as alcohol, caffeine withdrawal, sensory stimuli, certain food or food additives, medications, or changes in sleeping patterns. There may also be a genetic component to the prevalence of migraines, as they often run in families.

Most of the symptoms of these throbbing headaches, such as nausea and aversion to light or sound, are due to increased excitation of the trigeminovascular system, resulting in dilated blood vessels and neural inflammation. The subjective sensation of an 'aura' that often precedes a migraine has been shown to be due to increased signaling with the neurotransmitter glutamate. CBD has been shown to reduce this signaling. In fact, migraines are the most common condition treated by medical cannabis according to ancient and historical medical texts.

While there is no specific cure for migraines, there are many treatment options, such as dietary modification, and the addition of certain medications, such as pain relievers and triptans, that may help to relieve or reduce severity of symptoms. There are a variety of home remedies and alternative ideas for preventing, treating, and reducing the effects of migraines, which I will cover later in the chapter.

Studies have shown that people who suffer from migraines or chronic headaches are highly susceptible to other conditions such as anxiety, depression, chronic pain disorders, and epilepsy.

Migraine Symptoms:

- Aura
- Nausea
- Light/sound sensitivity
- Throbbing/pulsating pain
- Vision changes
- Pain on one side of head
- Vomiting
- Stiff neck

- Dizziness
- Weakness

CBD and Migraines

Dr. Ethan Russo, one of the leading scientists in the field of cannabinoid medications, believes that migraines, like fibromyalgia and irritable bowel syndrome (IBS), are due to a deficiency of the body's natural cannabinoids. According to his theory, increasing the body's level of natural cannabinoids by using CBD will help to reduce the occurrence of migraines.[28]

In a study done in Europe, researchers gave volunteers suffering from chronic migraines oral doses of a combination of THC and CBD. Once an oral dose of 400mg CBD/THC was administered, the acute pain caused by the migraines dropped by 55%. Phase II of the study found very similar results; after three months, cannabinoids reduced pain among migraine patients by 43.5%. Some patients did experience drowsiness as a result of the oral dosage of THC/CBD, but otherwise, the side effects were positive.[29, 30]

CBD can reduce the occurrence and severity of the episodes, so it is used as a preventive medicine; however, due to its long-acting mechanism, CBD is not generally used to control the acute onset of pain associated with migraines or non-migraine headaches. The slow onset of action of CBD and lack of efficacy for acute pain make CBD a poor choice for treating acute onset headaches and migraines. There are many safe and effective over-the-counter medications to treat acute onset headache and migraine pain.

CBD Extract:

Starting adult dose (not recommended in children): 5mg/dose of CBD extract under the tongue in the morning, afternoon, and at bedtime, for a total of 30mg a day.

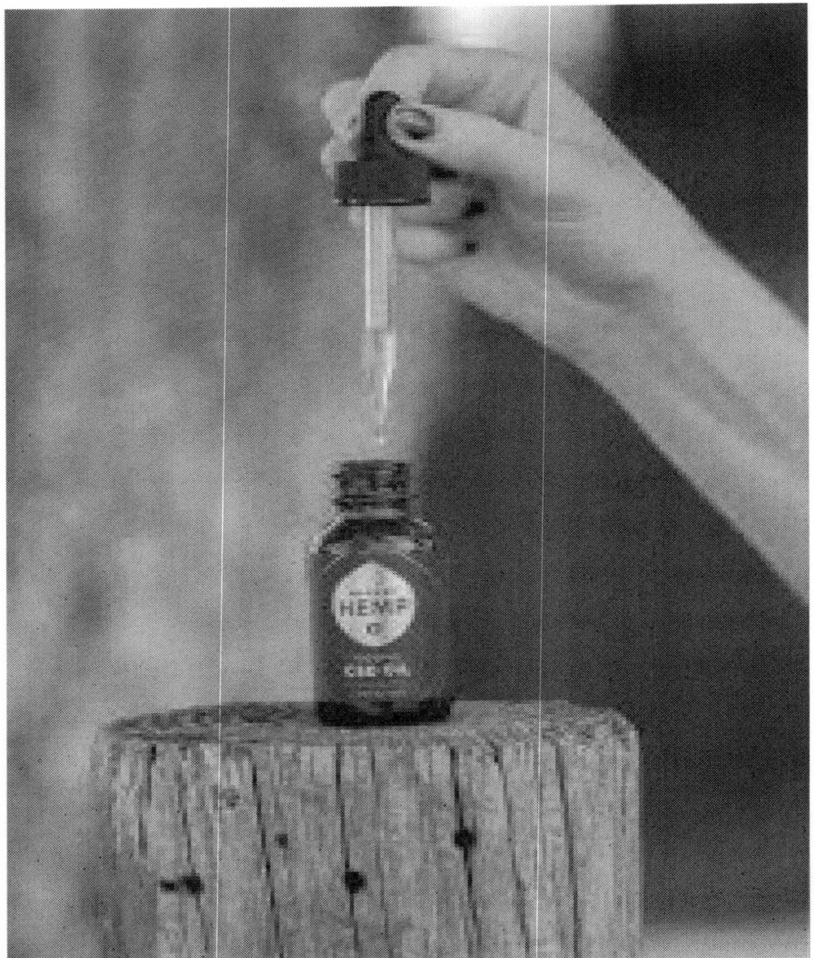

The dose may be increased by 5mg per dose, three times a day, every 4-5 days, depending on one's response to the medication; once maximum relief has been achieved with a certain dose, that dose should be maintained. Maximum daily dose is 200mg.

Treatment doesn't always work

Medicine is an art more than it is a science. Sometimes the recommended treatment doesn't work. It may not work because the dose wasn't correct, or it may not work because the underlying condition causing the symptoms is more severe than originally thought.

Start out with the recommended CBD extract dose and slowly work your way up; if the maximum doses of CBD extract isn't providing enough relief, it is time to go back to your physician for some advice.

Involving Medical Professionals

Chronic headaches can be very serious and debilitating on their own, or may represent a more serious underlying condition. Starting CBD for headache prevention should be considered only after discussion with your neurologist or primary-care physician. As is unfortunately usually the case, most physicians will have very little knowledge of CBD or medical marijuana, much less their potential use in headache prevention. Therefore, it is important to give your doctor the opportunity to assist in finding an effective means of controlling your headaches. Do not attempt to suddenly decrease or discontinue your prescription medications on your own. Involve your doctor while you gradually titrate the dose of CBD to control your headaches.

Chapter 8: Gastrointestinal Conditions

Colitis, Crohn's disease, Celiac disease, inflammatory bowel disease (IBD) and irritable bowel syndrome (IBS) are all disorders that affect the small and/ or large intestine. It is important to understand the difference between colitis and Crohn's disease versus IBS: Colitis and Crohn's disease are considered inflammatory bowel diseases (IBD), but Irritable Bowel Syndrome (IBS) does not fall into this category.

Relief of constipation was one of the original cannabis indications cited in Shen-Nung, 5,000 years ago, and cannabinoids have since been shown to have a variety of uses in the treatment of digestive problems. Cannabinoids are anti-spasmodic, relaxing and soothing tense muscles. They can also help with diarrhea by reducing inflammation in the intestinal wall.

Inflammatory Bowel Disease (IBD)

Colitis, which can be caused by infections or other diseases including Crohn's disease, is an inflammation of the inner lining of the colon. The colon is a hollow muscular tube that processes waste products delivered from higher up in the small intestine. It also removes water and eliminates the remnants as feces. When a person has colitis or Crohn's disease, the inner lining of this muscular tube becomes inflamed.

Colitis is considered common, with over 200,000 US cases a year, whereas Crohn's disease is a specific type of autoimmune disease and is rarer. Colitis affects people of all ages, but the majority of cases are seen in people ages 18-60; the majority of Crohn's disease cases are seen in people ages 19-40.

Both colitis and Crohn's disease patients are at increased risk for colon cancer and should be screened regularly by a physician. There is currently no cure for colitis or Crohn's disease, so most treatments are focused on relieving symptoms.

Colitis Symptoms:

- Abdominal pain
- Diarrhea
- Bloody stool
- Crohn's Disease Symptoms:
- Abdominal pain
- Diarrhea
- Weight loss
- Fatigue
- Anemia
- Celiac Symptoms:
- Diarrhea
- Bloating
- Gas
- Fatigue
- Low Blood Count

Irritable Bowel Syndrome (IBS)

IBS is an intestinal disorder that affects the colon causing various symptoms. There isn't a single known cause of IBS, but it is thought that a variety of factors impact the disorder. Fortunately, it does not put patients at higher risk for colon cancer.

Medical experts believe that some of the symptoms of IBS are caused by faulty communication between the brain and the intestinal tract. According to Mayo Clinic, the "walls of the intestines are lined with layers of muscle that contract and relax in a coordinated rhythm as they move food from your stomach through your intestinal tract to your rectum. If you have irritable bowel syndrome, the contractions may be stronger and last longer than normal, causing gas, bloating and diarrhea. Or the opposite may occur, with weak intestinal contractions slowing food passage and leading to hard, dry stools."[31]

IBS is considered a common disorder, with about 1 in 6 people in the US affected by symptoms at some time in their life. It also affects women twice as much as men, possibly due to hormonal changes in the menstrual cycle. While the disorder can affect people of all ages, it is most common in teen years through the 40's.

There is currently no cure for IBS, but through self-care and therapy, many patients are able to manage their symptoms. Changes in diet, exercise, and stress management can all reduce the severity of IBS and medications such as anti-diarrheals and laxatives may provide some symptom relief.

IBS Symptoms:

- Abdominal pain
- Cramping
- Bloated feeling
- Gas

- Constipation
- Diarrhea
- Mucus in the stool

The intestinal tract, including the small and large intestine, contains high levels of CB2 receptors. Use of CBD that stimulates these receptors will result in a positive therapeutic benefit related to muscle contraction (colicky pain) and absorption of water in the stool (diarrhea or constipation.) The high prevalence of CB2 receptors in the intestinal tract also means that CBD will turn down the inflammatory processes that cause colitis and Crohn's disease.

As with fibromyalgia and migraine headaches, Dr. Ethan Russo feels that IBS is due to a deficiency of the body's natural cannabinoids. According to his theory, increasing the body's level of natural cannabinoids by using CBD will reduce or resolve the symptoms of IBS. In the study, he found that CBD demonstrated the ability to block gastrointestinal mechanisms that promote symptoms of IBS, celiac disease, and other related disorders.

CBD Treatment

Considering that there aren't any specific cures for colitis, Crohn's disease or IBS, research into potential treatments for these conditions is ongoing. De Filippis et al. studied the effect of CBD on intestinal biopsies of patients with colitis, and from intestinal segments of mice with intestinal inflammation. In the conclusion of their study, they found:

"The results of the present study correlate and expand the findings suggesting CBD as a potent compound that is able to modulate experimental gut inflammation...in this study we demonstrate that during intestinal inflammation, CBD is able to control the inflammatory scenario and the subsequent intestinal apoptosis through the restoration of the altered glia-immune homeostasis. CBD is therefore regarded as a promising therapeutic agent that modulates the neuro-immune axis, which can be recognized as a new target in the treatment of inflammatory bowel disorders."[32]

Colitis, Crohn's disease and IBS all involve inflammation or irregular muscle movements and issues with water absorption in the large intestine, causing discomfort and a variety of symptoms. CBD increases the tone of the ECS. The gastrointestinal tract has large numbers of CB2 receptors. Activation of these CB2 receptors occurs through indirect effects of CBD. This reduces inflammation and promotes muscle relaxation, providing relief of symptoms such as cramps, diarrhea, constipation, and spasms.

CBD rectal suppositories are absorbed directly into the bloodstream in the very vascular rectal area. The available information suggests that between 50-70% of the CBD is absorbed directly into the bloodstream from rectal suppositories; this is far superior to the percent of CBD that is absorbed through the GI tract. Because these CBD suppositories do not go through the first-pass effect of the liver, the CBD may also have more local effects in the colon that are not available from oromucosal absorption. For these reasons, CBD rectal suppositories may be more effective than oromucosal absorption.

However, no research has been done to support the use of rectal suppositories over oromucosal absorption. Rectal suppositories only come in one dosage, 50mg. Therefore, it is difficult to gradually titrate a dose of a rectal suppository like you can with oil extracts. The price of suppositories is much higher per dose than an oil extract. Furthermore, three times daily of insertion of a rectal suppository with a latex glove may not be an attractive option for many people.

Dosing

CBD Extract: Starting adult dose (not recommended in children): 10mg of CBD extract under the tongue (oromuscosal absorption), morning, afternoon and bedtime. May increase by 10mg every 4-5 days, depending on response to the medication. Once maximum pain relief has been achieved with a certain dose, maintain that dose. Maximum daily dose 200mg. If there is not optimal relief of symptoms with the ‘maximum daily dose’ then stop the oromucosal route and try using rectal suppositories (below.)

Rectal suppository: Starting adult dose (not recommended for children) is one suppository (50mg CBD) inserted into the rectum with a latex glove three times daily: once in the morning, in the afternoon, and at bedtime.

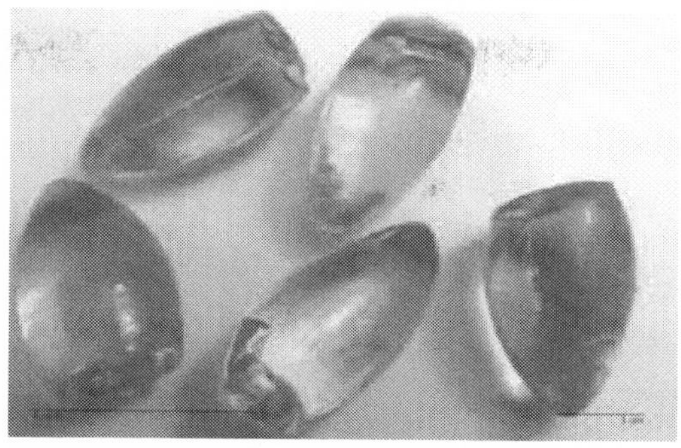

Treatment doesn't always work

Medicine is an art, more than it is a science. Sometimes the recommended treatment doesn't work. It may not work because the combination of medications wasn't correct, or it may not work because the underlying condition causing the symptoms is more severe than originally thought. Start out with just CBD extract. If the maximum doses of CBD extract and the rectal suppositories are not getting you enough relief, it is time to go back to your physician for further guidance.

Involving Medical Professionals:

IBS and Celiac disease are not life-threatening conditions, but they can seriously impact a person's quality of life. Trying CBD extract or suppositories to treat these conditions is generally quite safe, and may be very effective. Colitis and Crohn's diseases are serious inflammatory conditions of the bowel, so adding CBD should be considered only after discussion with your gastroenterologist or primary care physician. As is unfortunately usually the case, most physicians will have very little knowledge of CBD or medical marijuana, let alone their use in colitis and Crohn's disease. However, it is important to give your doctor the opportunity to assist you controlling your colitis symptoms. Do not attempt to suddenly decrease or discontinue your prescription medications. Involve your doctor, while you gradually titrate the dose of CBD to control your condition.

Chapter 9: Arthritis

Arthritis is the chronic inflammation of one or more joints, causing stiffness and pain in the tissues that surround the joints. According to the CDC, more than 54 million American adults have some form of arthritis, and about 32 million of those adults are of working age. It is important to note that arthritis does not refer to a single disease per se, but is an informal way of referring to general joint pain or joint disease. There are currently more than 100 types of arthritis and similarly related conditions. Some of the more common types of arthritis include degenerative, inflammatory, autoimmune, infectious, and metabolic.

Arthritis Symptoms:

- Pain
- Stiffness
- Reduced range of motion
- Swelling

The symptoms caused by arthritis vary from person to person and even day-by-day. For some patients, arthritis symptoms may come and go and vary from mild to severe; for others, the symptoms may stay stable over a few years, or get worse over time. Not only is arthritis painful, but it can cause permanent joint changes, and be so severe that the pain results in an inability to do daily activities.

The diagnosis of arthritis usually begins with a primary care physician to help determine the type of arthritis. If the arthritis is inflammatory or due to an autoimmune disease a rheumatologist, or medical specialist in arthritis, is usually seen. Depending on the severity of the arthritis. sometimes orthopedic surgery, such as joint replacements, will be required. There is currently no cure for arthritis, and just as with the symptoms, there is a large variety of treatments used. Strategies such as weight loss and exercise, physical therapies like massage and stretching, replacement surgeries, and medications such as anti-inflammatories, steroid and pain creams, are all current treatments for arthritis.

CBD Treatment

As mentioned above, arthritis is characterized by inflammation of the joints. In a study done by Dr. Sheng-Ming Dai, it was found that CB2 receptors are found in unusually high levels in the joint tissue of arthritis patients.[33] The use of cannabis is shown to fight inflammation in the joints by activating the pathways of CB2 receptors. These high levels of CB2 receptors are not present on healthy tissues, so the cells in the inflamed area results in increased production of CB2 receptors to help modify or reduce the local inflammation.

In another study conducted by Malfait et al., they used mice with collagen-induced arthritis. The CBD was administered orally and injected into the mice after the onset of arthritis symptoms. They found that 5 mg/kg per day injected and 25 mg/kg per day taken orally produced the most optimal effect. The study concluded that CBD was effective in both the prevention of joint damage and the treatment of arthritis.[34]

Osteoarthritis is a type of arthritis characterized as a degenerative joint disease with cartilage degradation. Currently, there are no drugs or treatments to control the progression of this disease. However, there is increasing evidence that the endocannabinoid system (ECS) may be a therapeutic target for the pain created by osteoarthritis. In preclinical studies done with rodent models with osteoarthritis, there is evidence suggesting that the ECS plays a role in the functional changes of osteoarthritis. While there is limited clinical evidence at the moment, preclinical studies indicate that cannabinoids such as CBD could play an important role in treating osteoarthritis symptoms.

There is quite a bit of evidence in animals showing that CBD is effective for arthritis. The Arthritis Society is currently funding grants for further research in the relationships between cannabinoids and arthritis and many other studies are being conducted on the topic, which will hopefully provide answers and relief for people suffering from arthritis.

There are several goals of treatment: to decrease pain, decrease swelling, stiffness and inflammation and finally to prevent the progression of the damage to the joints. The chapter on chronic pain provides a good discussion of how to use CBD, PEA, and acetaminophen to treat chronic arthritic pain. Since CBD decreases the body's inflammatory response, it also results in decreased swelling, stiffness, and inflammation of the joint. Finally, many cases of arthritis, such as RA and lupus, are due to autoimmune conditions. When there is an autoimmune condition, the body's immune system is attacking the normal cells in the lining of the joints. Since CBD modulates this autoimmune response, treatment can actually help prevent progression of the disease, not just treat the symptoms.

The newer 'biologic drugs' advertised heavily on TV and long-term use of steroid medications have been associated with severe and sometimes life-threatening side effects. By modulating the body's immune and inflammatory responses, CBD, dosed correctly, can help you and your doctor decrease or discontinue dosing these hazardous medications.

Some arthritis is limited to one joint, such as gout, or post-traumatic arthritis. Many times, an arthritic condition causes joint swelling and pain in easy-to-reach areas such as the hands, knees or shoulders. In these cases, topical application of CBD balms, in combination with over-the-counter creams containing camphor, salicylate, menthol and capsaicin should be tried. The topical treatment can be tried by itself, or in combination with CBD extracts under the tongue.

Dosing for all forms of arthritis

CBD Extract:_Starting adult dose (not recommended in children) is 10mg of CBD extract under the tongue three times daily, once in the morning, once in the afternoon, and again at bedtime.

The dose may be increased by 10mg every 4-5 days, depending on one's response to the medication, with a maximum daily dose of 200mg. Once maximum pain relief has been achieved with a certain dose, that dose should be maintained. Topical CBD balm can be applied to swollen, inflamed joints three times daily.

Treatment doesn't always work

Medicine is an art, more than it is a science. Sometimes the recommended treatment doesn't work. It may not work because the combination of medications wasn't correct, or it may not work because the underlying condition causing the pain, swelling or stiffness is more severe than originally thought. Start out with just CBD topicals and/or extract. If the maximum doses of CBD is not providing enough symptom relief, it is time to go back to your physician for some advice.

Involving Medical Professionals

Arthritis can be a simple age or trauma-related chronic condition, or it can be a serious, and sometimes life-threatening condition. The medications that are prescribed for inflammatory forms of arthritis are also serious and need to be managed by a physician. Always involve your rheumatologist or treating physician with decisions to add CBD or medical cannabis to the treatment of arthritis. Sometimes CBD alone is not enough to get control of the pain, and strains of medical marijuana containing THC are required.

Chapter 10:
Acne, Psoriasis and Other Skin Conditions

Personal Story

A lovely gentleman came in to see me with very red, scaly, large patches of psoriasis on his knees and elbows. He was distraught because he loved to wear shorts and a t-shirt in the warm California climate, but he felt ugly with the large red plaques on the front of his knees and back of his elbows. He had tried several medicated creams, without much effect. He did not want to have the severe side-effects that can occur with the potent and expensive biologic medications that are advertised on TV.

After a detailed history and exam, I found that he was an excellent candidate to use topical medical cannabis. Psoriasis is an inherited condition, caused by excess build-up of skin cells, and causes ugly raised red patches, that are often itchy and painful. I started him on a twice-daily preparation of CBD and THC cannabis cream. Because the inflamed surface of his skin would more easily absorb medication into the bloodstream than healthy skin, I warned him not to apply too much to the skin. He returned six weeks later wearing a t-shirt, shorts and a big smile on his face.

Introduction

The skin is the largest organ of the body. It is made of several layers, each with a different type of cell. It also has glands that produce sweat, and hair follicles connected with glands that produce oily sebum. At the base of the layers of the skin are the cells that produce protective pigment, called melanocytes. These are when melanoma cancer starts.

Skin Condition Symptoms:

- Rash
- Peeling skin
- Ulcers
- Raised bumps
- Discolored patches of skin
- Dry or cracked skin
- Open Sores
- Rough or scaly skin

CBD Treatment

The skin cells, called keratocytes, have both CB1 and CB2 receptors; the hair follicle has only CB1 receptors, while the sebaceous glands and subcutaneous tissue cells have only CB2 receptors. TRPV1 receptors are found in the tiny skin nerve fibers and send the sensation of itchiness or burning to the brain.

In general, patients try topical CBD preparations because regular medications are not working, as was the case with the gentleman in my story. Another good reason to try topical cannabis is that some prescription medications may have severe side effects. As you will learn, topical cannabis has only a few mild side effects, all of which resolve by discontinuing the medication.

The term 'pruritus' means itching that can occur anywhere on the body. This can be caused by bug bites, healing wounds, dry skin, or a variety of skin conditions. A study was done by S Stander, et al. with 22 patients experiencing itching of the skin. They were given a topical cannabinoid in the form of a cream to reduce the itching. The results of the study showed that the reduction in itching was 86.4% after the topical cream was used. The researchers concluded that topical cannabinoids, such as CBD, represent a well-tolerated and effective treatment for the reduction of itching in various conditions.[35, 36]

CBD has also been proven to have anti-inflammatory properties, which is useful in the treatment of certain types of skin conditions such as acne vulgaris.[37] Inflammatory acne is caused by chronic inflammation of the skin, and CBD can reduce the inflammation around pimples, which decrease the likelihood of acne spreading. However, stimulation of CB2 receptors in the follicles can also increase the amount of sebum being produced, which would aggravate the acne. CBD has also been shown to have antioxidant effects, which can protect the skin from free radicals such as smoke, oils, and UV rays; protecting the skin from these radicals can help prevent and treat various skin conditions.

The skin has many functions; it provides protection against ultraviolet light and a physical barrier that prevents chemicals and microbes from entering the body. It has several other functions related to the production of moisturizing sebum, and regulation of the body's temperature through sweat release and hair. Underneath the skin layer is the subcutaneous tissue that is very fibrotic in nature; several conditions can result in excess fibrosis tissue formation. The following are common skin conditions that can be treated with CBD with promising results.

Acne is a very common skin condition, especially in teenagers and in some adults, with over 3 million cases a year in the US. It occurs when hair follicles plug with oil and dead skin cells, and it can occur anywhere on the body. According to the American Academy of Dermatology, acne is the most common skin conditions in the United States.

Psoriasis is another very common skin condition that affects over 3 million Americans a year, is characterized by the buildup of skin cells into dry, itchy patches and scales. Unlike acne, psoriasis is an autoimmune disease. It is treatable, but unfortunately not curable. The areas most commonly affected by psoriasis are the knees, scalp, and outside of elbows, but it can occur anywhere on the body. There are various severities of psoriasis.

Psoriasis is due to excess proliferation of the top layer of cells, known as keratocytes. The keratocytes have both CB1 and CB2 receptors. Cannabis-infused topical medications will decrease how fast these cells are reproducing or proliferating, and increase the rate of programmed cell suicide, called apoptosis. The CBD, since it impacts the THCV1 receptor, will decrease the perception of itch, heat and pain that often accompanies thick psoriatic plaques.

Eczema and **atopic or irritant dermatitis** are due to inflammation in the skin layers in response to allergens or chemical irritants. In addition to red, irritated skin, eczema is often accompanied by an itching, burning sensation. It responds nicely to a CBD topical, which activates CB1, CB2 and TRPV1. This results in decreased inflammation and swelling, and decreased perception of itch, heat and pain.

Sunburn is just a variation of dermatitis, defined as inflammation and swelling in the skin due to excessive sun exposure. Skin cells typically have both CB1 and CB2 receptors, and cannabis can be used as a preventive to decrease the damage from UVB light and inflammation and swelling after excess sun exposure. However, the use of 30+ sunblock, protective clothing, and decreasing sun or artificial UVB light exposure are primary means of preventing skin cancers and sunburn.

Insect bites result in localized inflammation and burning sensations via the TRPV1 receptors. CBD often erases these effects immediately.

Fibrosis in the subcutaneous tissues can cause conditions such as scleroderma, Peyronie's disease of the shaft of the penis, and Dupuytren's contractures of the hand or feet (below). These tissues only have CB2 receptors. Stimulation of the CB2 receptor leads to decreased inflammation and fibrotic tissue formation.

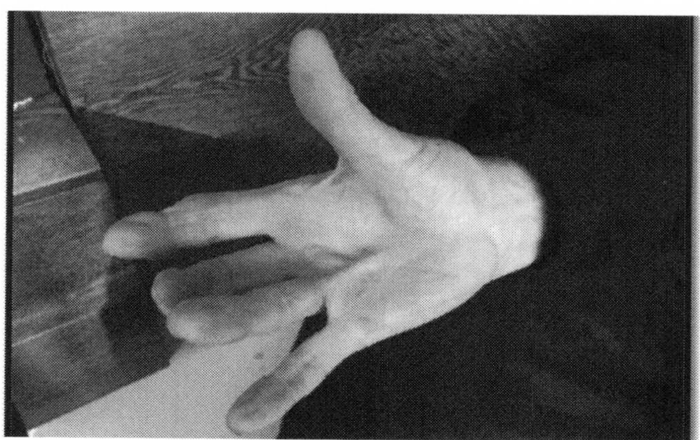

Hair loss is usually due to decreased hair shaft elongation, and the hair follicle going dormant. The hair follicle has CB1 receptors; unfortunately, activation of CB1 on the hair follicle results in decreased hair shaft growth, causing the follicle to go dormant. Therefore, no cannabis-infused topical preparation is currently recommended.

More than any other condition listed above, skin cancer (basal cell, squamous cell, or melanoma) needs to be treated under the strict supervision of a medical provider. While cannabis-infused medications may be a helpful addition to the treatment, the available evidence does not support using cannabis alone to treat skin cancer.

Considering there are so many different types of skin conditions with different underlying causes, there is also a variety of potential treatments for such conditions, some of which may be more effective for some than others. Acne, for example, can be treated with oral antibiotics, medicated soaps, topical retinoids, lotions, or contraceptives in women; Psoriasis, an autoimmune condition, is often treated with steroid creams, light therapy, vitamin D, or biological drugs. Other skin conditions can be managed by drugs, topical creams or soaps, and paying close attention to one's individual lifestyle choices, such as diet and exercise.

Dosing

CBD has long-acting effects, so initially, try using the topical preparation once a day in a thick layer. Gently rub the medication into the skin to improve penetration into the tissues. Depending on what condition you are treating, give the once-a-day application a chance to work for 5-7 days before considering going to twice a day. If, after two weeks of regular application you are not getting satisfactory results, consider buying a different product with a higher strength of CBD, or different vehicle in the preparation. Usually, the less expensive and more popular brands will have less CBD in them than more expensive products. Don't stop taking any topical medications prescribed by your doctor without consulting in advance.

There are several conditions where subcutaneous, or under the skin, fibrotic nodules result in a painful or impairing condition, or disfigurement. Dupuytren's contracture of the hand (shown in the photo above) and Peyronie's disease, which is a fibrotic contracture of the base of the penis, both respond very nicely to CBD topical. Scleroderma is an autoimmune disease that results in a serious condition due to increased fibroblast cell activity in several organs. This also responds to long-term use of CBD. Fibroblast cells, which many CB2 receptors on them, form these scar-like tissue under the skin. Activation of the CB2 receptors with CBD results in decreased tissue fibrosis in the skin and organs, such as the liver.

Dosing Fibrotic Nodules

For treatment of one to a few subcutaneous nodules, local application of CBD twice daily for 2-3 weeks usually results in marked reduction in nodule size, thickness and symptoms. To improve the penetration of the CBD into nodule, it is recommended that a thick portion of high-potency CBD gel or cream is used. A latex or similar glove is placed over the hand or penis; the glove seals the medicine in, resulting in deeper absorption into the subcutaneous tissues.

Dosing for Scleroderma or Liver Fibrosis

The goal for CBD treatment for these chronic conditions is to maintain an increased level of CB2 activation on fibroblast cells throughout the skin and organs of the body. So the treatment is 20mg three times daily, ongoing. The dose can be increased after 60 days to 30mg three times daily, if there is no effect from 20mg dose. Keep increasing the dose by 10mg, every 60 days up to maximum of 200mg.

Other ingredients

For the skin conditions in this chapter, purchase a CBD topical that doesn't have added ingredients for muscles or joints. Many other ingredients can be added to topical medications including cayenne, camphor, capsaicin, clove, wintergreen, and menthol. Most of these are essential oils that have been used for hundreds of years for topical application for sore muscles and stiffness. These ingredients are added when the topical preparation is being used for a local joint or muscle pain or swelling, and not for the skin conditions described in this chapter.

Treatment doesn't always work

Medicine is an art, more than it is a science. Sometimes the recommended treatment doesn't work. It may not work because the dose wasn't correct, or it may not work because the underlying condition causing the symptoms is more severe than originally thought.

Involving Medical Professionals

Skin conditions can be serious, and sometimes represent a more serious underlying condition in the body. Many skin conditions need to be managed by a physician. Always involve your treating physician with decisions to add CBD or medical cannabis to the treatment of serious or chronic skin conditions.

Chapter 11:
Seizures and Epilepsy

Personal story

A concerned mother of a child with epilepsy and autism came to see me. She was visiting from Georgia and wanted to get a medical marijuana card. She was going to use the card to get medical marijuana for her daughter and bring it back to Georgia. I examined her daughter and determined that her autism and epilepsy had a good chance of responding to CBD. I told her she didn't need a medical marijuana card because she could get all of the high-quality CBD oil she needed mailed directly to her home in Atlanta, and gave her my personal recommendations.

She felt a little silly for driving seven hours each way to find that out, so I didn't charge her for the consultation. I told her to make certain that the pediatrician in Atlanta was involved with her care. A few months later, I received a nice email from her where she thanked me for my advice and happily reported to me that her daughter's autism and epilepsy symptoms had responded wonderfully after just a few months of treatment with CBD oil, and that the child was doing great.

Introduction

A seizure happens when there are changes in the brain's electrical activity. Brain cells inhibit or excite other brain cells from sending messages and while there is usually a balance of these cells, during a seizure there is too much or too little activity, causing an imbalance. These imbalances can lead to chemical changes in the brain which cause a surge of electrical activity, resulting in the seizure.

There are a variety of types of seizures, including non-epileptic, partial, and generalized. Non-epileptic seizures are usually caused by a head trauma, and often go away once the condition is treated. Some seizures result in mild symptoms, whereas severe seizures can lead to violent shaking and loss of control. As you can see from the "Symptoms" list, not all epileptic seizures result in dramatic movements of the arms and legs. Sometimes the seizure activity in the brain just results in an "aura", or sensation that something abnormal is happening, resulting in staring spells.

Epilepsy is the diagnosis when someone has a condition that results in recurrent seizures. It is a central nervous system condition in which nerve cell activity in the brain is disturbed, causing seizures. Epilepsy, or seizure disorder, affects three million Americans. While any age group can be affected by epilepsy, the majority of new diagnoses are in children. The causes of epilepsy vary and can include a specific problem in the brain causing the seizures, but more than half of epilepsy cases in children are idiopathic, meaning they have no clear cause or obvious problem in the brain. There are several genetic causes of epilepsy, especially the very severe, intractable forms of infantile and childhood epilepsy.

To diagnose epilepsy, a doctor will inquire about symptoms, and may order tests such as an electroencephalogram (EEG) to measure electrical activity of the brain, or magnetic resonance imaging (MRI) to look at images of the brain. At this time, there is no cure for epilepsy, only treatments. Medicine to prevent the seizures is usually the first line of treatment to manage epilepsy, but a special diet or very rarely implantation of a nerve stimulator have also been used to treat the disorder.

Unfortunately, in over 30% of the cases, even multiple prescription medications don't adequately control the seizures, and in another significant proportion of the patients, the side effects from their prescription medications are so bad that the patient can't take the medication. Adult-onset seizure disorder is usually due to direct head trauma, or other more clearly recognized conditions. However, just as with younger sufferers of epilepsy, many adults have problems maintaining control of their seizures with the available prescription medications.

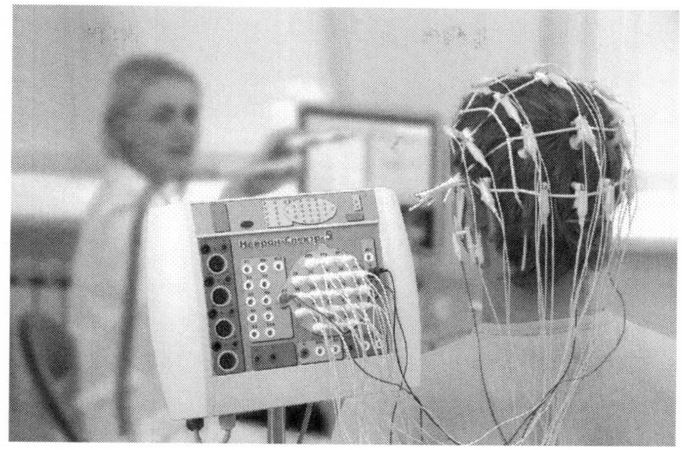

The widespread acceptance of the use of CBD for treating infantile seizures began in 2009, after the Stanley Brothers began breeding a high-CBD strain of cannabis specifically for the treatment of seizure disorder. This strain was eventually named "Charlotte's Web" in 2012 after Charlotte Figi had dramatic success with using CBD to control her intractable seizures. Subsequently, the Realm of Caring (www.theROC.us) was started to provide assistance to these devastated families and children. I strongly recommend this website for anyone considering CBD or medical marijuana for their child with epilepsy. In addition to a patient-focused newsletter, they have local workshops and "care specialist consultations." They also have discounts for "Charlotte's Web" CBD formulations. The products from www.CWhemp.com have my highest recommendation.

FDA-Approved Seizure Drugs

The only two conditions for which the CBD isolate Epidiolex® has been granted FDA approval are the two rare intractable pediatric seizure disorders: Dravet's syndrome (DS) and Lennox-Gastaut syndrome (LGS). The recommended starting dose is 10mg/kg maintenance dose up to a maximum of 20mg/kg a day. That would be 800-1600mg a day for an 80-kilogram person. This exceptionally high dose is due to the fact that Epidiolex® was studied as an ingested oral solution, and 90% of it is turned into inactive metabolites via the first-pass effect. The individual annual cost of this treatment in the US comes to around $32,500.

In placebo-controlled trials of patients with LGS or DS, 323 patients received Epidiolex® for up to 14 weeks. Approximately 46% of patients were female, 83% were Caucasian, and the mean age was 14 years (range 2 to 48 years). All patients were taking other seizure medications. In controlled trials, the rate of discontinuation as a result of any adverse reaction was 2.7% for patients taking Epidiolex® 10 mg/kg/day, 11.8% for patients taking Epidiolex® 20 mg/kg/day, and 1.3% for patients on placebo. The most frequent cause of discontinuations was liver function elevation. Discontinuation for liver function elevation occurred at an incidence of 1.3% in patients taking Epidiolex® 10 mg/kg/day, 5.9% in patients taking Epidiolex® 20 mg/kg/day, and 0.4% in patients on placebo.[38]

Somnolence, sedation, and lethargy were among the major side effects which ultimately led to discontinuation among 3% of patients taking Epidiolex® 20 mg/kg/day, compared to 0% of patients taking Epidiolex® 10 mg/kg/day or on placebo. The most common adverse reactions that occurred in Epidiolex®-treated patients (incidence at least 10% and greater than placebo) were somnolence, decreased appetite, diarrhea, transaminase elevations, fatigue, malaise, and asthenia, rash, insomnia, sleep disorders, poor quality sleep, and infections.[39]

Seizures

Up to 35% of patients, both adults and children, with refractory epilepsy have inadequate seizure control, despite currently available drugs. In addition, seizure medications tend to come with significant side effects. Because of this, there has been growing interest in the use of CBD for the treatment of medically refractory epilepsy. This need, combined with recent media attention focused on the benefits of CBD in the treatment of refractory epilepsy, has spurred a series of clinical trials in an attempt to more clearly understand the risks and benefits associated with this treatment for a variety seizure types

Even after the FDA approval of Epidiolex®, the drug's exact mechanism of action is not fully understood. In addition to CBD's effects on the ECS, CBD is a very promiscuous molecule, having been shown to act on multiple other receptors outside of the ECS, which play a key role in seizure activity. CBD is thought to inhibit synaptic transmission of electrical activity and to raise the seizure threshold via CB1 receptors and other non-ECS receptors.[40] There are several studies showing the efficacy of CBD for other forms of intractable pediatric and adult epilepsy.[41, 42, 43] Studies have shown CBD to have anti-seizure effects through the same mechanisms discussed above.

CBD Treatment

Intractable epilepsy refers to a condition that cannot be adequately controlled by medication. About 30% of children and adults diagnosed with epilepsy are not able to gain control of the seizures with the available FDA-approved medications. Inherited conditions, such as Dravet's, usually cause intractable epilepsy, but many non-inherited causes of epilepsy are also unable to be controlled with up to 12 different FDA-approved epilepsy drugs.

CBD has been shown to be moderately to highly effective at reducing frequency and severity of seizures. In a small study of treatment-resistant epileptic children, some of whom had a specific condition, and others who had idiopathic epilepsy, the use of CBD was found to be effective in 16 of the 19 children;[44] The average number of antiepileptic drugs each child had tried prior to the CBD treatment was 12.

In this study, 14 parents reported seizure reduction in their children, and 2 reported their child's seizures stopping altogether. They also described other beneficial effects such as better mood, improved sleep, and increased alertness. These findings correlate with another major study at epilepsy treatment centers worldwide which showed that patients who received CBD treatment experienced a 45.1 percent reduction in seizures.[43]

In a study done by Dr. Robert DeLorenzo, his team found that cannabinoids effectively decreased seizures by activating the brain's CB1 receptors. The study indicates that "cannabinoids may offer unique advantages in treating seizures compared with currently prescribed seizure medications... Ingredients in marijuana and the cannabinoid receptor protein produced naturally in the body to regulate the central nervous system and other bodily functions play a critical role in controlling spontaneous seizures in epilepsy."[45]

Based upon the research, it's clear that CBD has had positive effects on reducing seizures in children and adults with epilepsy, but this is a fairly new discovery, offering room for further research and a better understanding of the relationship between CBD and epilepsy.

THC is sometimes present in "High-CBD" products. THC, however, can actually aggravate epilepsy, so make certain that the products you choose are certified laboratory-tested with a Certificate of Analysis (COA) showing that they contain very low amounts of THC (less than 0.3%).

Involving Medical Professionals

Childhood or adult-onset epilepsy is a significant and potentially life-threatening condition. It is possible that the large doses of CBD required to control seizures may change the liver enzymes metabolism of prescription drugs used to treat epilepsy. Due to the complexity and severity of seizure disorder, and possibility of medication interaction, patients and guardians of patients with epilepsy should always work closely with their neurologist to determine if adding CBD or medical marijuana is appropriate. Dosing and titration should be managed by the treating medical professional only.

Chapter 12: Fibromyalgia

Fibromyalgia (FM) is defined simply as chronic, widespread muscle tenderness and pain. It is a common disorder, impacting more than 3 million Americans a year. This disorder affects more women than men, and can happen to anyone of any age. Just as with many pain disorders, symptoms can vary in type and intensity from person to person, or even day to day.

Fibromyalgia Symptoms

- Fatigue
- Sleep disturbances
- Cognitive difficulties
- Stiffness
- Depression
- Anxiety
- Tension headaches
- Pelvic pain
- Bowel/bladder issues
- Migraines

While there is currently no known cause of FM, decades of research is allowing medical providers to begin to understand its potential contributing factors. Some of these possible factors include infections, trauma, genetics, and stress. There are different thoughts on what causes the pain experienced with FM- one theory suggests that the brain might lower the pain threshold, changing one's perception of pain. Another thought is that the receptors and nerves in the body become more sensitive to stimulation, overacting and causing exaggerated pain.

FM is similar to MS in that there isn't a single test to detect FM; instead, tests are done to rule out potential underlying causes of pain and other symptoms. Widespread pain that lasts for three months or longer, particularly pain that has no other identifiable cause, is usually the beginning of a FM diagnosis. Unfortunately, FM is a chronic condition, meaning that the majority of people diagnosed with the disorder will have it the rest of their lives.

There is no cure for FM. Therefore, doctors attempt to manage the pain and improve quality of life through medications. Pain relievers and antidepressants. Anti-seizure medications, such as Neurontin® and Lyrica®, are used because they stabilize nerves that send pain messages. There are alternative treatments for FM intended to be used in conjunction with medication, including acupuncture, physical therapy, yoga, meditation, massage therapy, diet, and regular exercise.

CBD Treatment

There are have been various studies done on the relationship between cannabis and FM symptoms. One study of FM patients done by J. Fiz et al. measured pain, stiffness, relaxation, and well-being in 28 cannabis users and 28 non-cannabis users.[46] The results found that after 2 hours of cannabis use, the users showed a statistically significant reduction of stiffness and pain, increased relaxation, and an increase feeling of well-being. The conclusion of this study was that cannabis was associated with beneficial effects on some FM symptoms. It is not clear how much of the effects are due to THC versus CBD.

Dr. Ethan Russo, one of the founding fathers of medical cannabis research, has postulated that FM is due to a deficiency of the body's endocannabinoids, much as depression is due to a deficiency of the body's serotonin. Since CBD enhances the level of natural endocannabinoids in the brain and body, this remedies the deficiency and reduces the body's response to painful stimuli. The elevated levels of natural cannabinoids also result in improved sleep and mood, both issues associated with FM.

Since FM is often accompanied by specific areas of the body that are very painful, both CBD taken orally and applied topically should be used. In FM, there is no actual injury or inflamed tissue or muscles; the problem is that the brain is perceiving pain throughout the body, so there is no need to actually treat any swelling or spasm. With FM, the "tender points" around the body are areas where slight pressure cause the sensation of unexpected or intense pain.

As we discussed above in the chronic pain chapter, PEA and acetaminophen are also helpful in reducing pain, thereby eliminating the need for muscle relaxants and addictive opioids.

Dosing

CBD Extract: Starting adult dose (not recommended in children) 10mg of CBD extract under the tongue, morning, afternoon and bedtime._May increase by 10mg every 4-5 days, depending on response to the medication. Once maximum pain relief has been achieved with a certain dose, maintain that dose. Maximum daily dose 200mg. PEA and acetaminophen can be taken at same times as CBD extract.

PEA Capsule: Starting adult dose (not recommended in children) 400mg capsule once a day. May increase after four days to 400mg twice a day, then up to three times a day, depending on response to the medication._Once maximum pain relief has been achieved with a certain dose, maintain that dose. Maximum daily dose 1400mg.

Acetaminophen: Starting adult dose (not recommended in children) is 625mg extended-release capsule three times a day. Prolonged or excessive use of acetaminophen can cause liver damage, and other conditions. This is especially true when using acetaminophen and alcoholic beverages. Always read the package insert and consult your physician if there is any question about the appropriate use of acetaminophen. Be careful to make certain that you are not getting acetaminophen (Tylenol®) in any other medications that you are taking.

The extended release version of Tylenol®, called "arthritis pain formula", lasts eight hours and provides a more consistent control of chronic pain- 3,000mg is maximum daily dose. This is the only dose recommended without consulting a physician.

Treatment doesn't always work

Medicine is an art more than it is a science. Sometimes the recommended treatment doesn't work. It may not work because the combination of medications wasn't correct, or it may not work because the underlying condition causing the pain is more severe than originally thought.

Start out with just CBD topicals and/or extract. If, after 2 weeks, you have not achieved a satisfactory level of pain relief, add acetaminophen. Give the acetaminophen at least a week to improve the pain; if you still have not reached the desired level, add the PEA capsules. If the maximum doses of these three medications are not getting you enough pain relief, it is time to go back to your physician for advice.

Involving Medical Professionals

As I stated before, in patients with FM, there is no actual injury or inflammation in the muscles or tissues; the increased perception of pain and the functional effects of this pain are the primary problem. As is, unfortunately, usually the case, most physicians will have very little knowledge of CBD, PEA or medical marijuana, and their use in chronic pain. However, it is important to give your doctor the opportunity to assist you controlling your FM. Do not attempt to suddenly decrease or discontinue your prescription medications. Involve your doctor and ask her to help you gently taper off the prescription medications, why you gradually titrate the dose of CBD and other medications discussed above.

Chapter 13:
Multiple Sclerosis, Spasm and Spasticity

I will begin this chapter with another relevant personal anecdote. A family friend of mine named Brian was suffering from a very advanced case of MS, and had been getting medical cannabis from a friend in California. He showed me his bottles of extracts, and said he wasn't noticing much effect and he was getting 'high' when he used the extract.

Upon further examination, it became apparent that the extract from California was very high in THC (20%), and very low in CBD. In other words, the extract was designed for recreational use, and was certainly not intended to treat MS. I directed Brian to a CBD manufacturer from which he could order legal, safe, high quality, pure CBD oil.

He only recently received it, so I have yet to hear back regarding how his MS has responded to the CBD, but in general MS patients report CBD having very positive effects on their burning pain, muscle and bladder spasms, and mood.

The important point is that just because it is from the marijuana plant doesn't necessarily mean it is medically appropriate to treat any condition. Most of the 'medical marijuana' for sale in California dispensaries is very high in THC and has almost no CBD. This is not going to treat anything but boredom. Get educated, know what you are buying, follow the dosing advice, and great things will happen.

Introduction

Multiple Sclerosis (MS) is a disease of the central nervous system in which the immune system eats away at the protective covering of nerves, known as myelin, similar to the plastic covering around copper wires. If this covering is removed, electrical signals are unable to transmit correctly. This type of nerve damage disrupts communication between the brain and the body, causing a variety of problems, some of which can be debilitating.

MS affects more than 2.3 million people worldwide. It is thought that there are less than 200,000 cases a year in the US, but because the CDC does not require physicians to report new cases and sometimes symptoms are invisible, these numbers are only an estimate, and may not be entirely accurate.

While symptoms present differently in each person who suffers from MS, some of the more common ones are listed below.

MS Symptoms:

- Fatigue
- Walking difficulties
- Spasticity (muscle stiffness)
- Muscle spasms
- Weakness
- Numbness or tingling
- Vision problems
- Bladder/bowel problems
- Pain
- Cognitive changes
- Depression

There is no specific known cause for MS, and there is also no specific test for the disease. However, MRI results can sometimes show issues in the brain or spinal cord. During the diagnostic process, a person can expect blood tests, a spinal tap, a MRI, and a test which records electrical signals produced by the nervous system. MS is a serious condition, so doctors usually first try to rule out other conditions that might explain the symptomatology.

Treatment is aimed at preventing progression of the attack on the myelin sheaths, managing the symptoms and speeding recovery from attacks. There are several existing treatments for MS, including corticosteroids, which are prescribed to reduce nerve inflammation. Plasma exchange is another treatment option, which involves removing the liquid portion of a person's blood (plasma) and separating it from the blood cells, which are then mixed with a protein and put back into the body. There is currently only one FDA-approved medication, Ocrevus®, which is used to slow the worsening of disability in people with primary-progressive MS.

For people with relapsing-remitting MS, there are many disease-modifying therapies used to attempt to treat the disease, but most of these options carry significant health risks. To treat the symptoms of MS, physical therapy, muscle relaxants, and medications to treat fatigue, depression, and pain are commonly used.

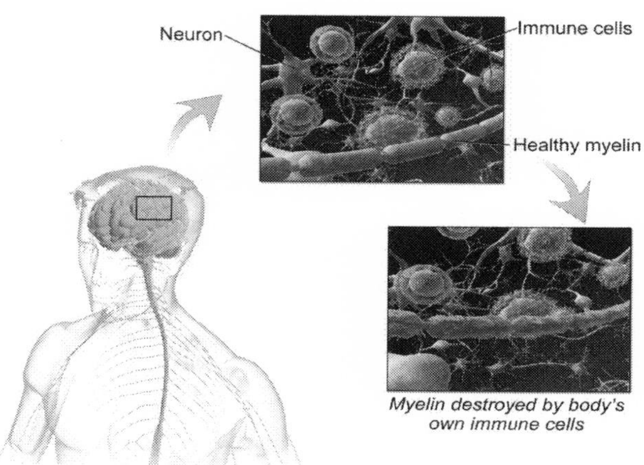

Many people try alternative medicine as a primary or a complementary treatment to help manage symptoms. Yoga, meditation, diet change, and exercise may boost overall physical and mental well-being, which, in turn, may provide some relief for MS symptoms.

CBD Treatment

Guidelines from the American Academy of Neurology recommend the use of oral cannabis extract for muscle spasticity and pain, but due to lack of research and evidence, they don't recommend cannabis in any other form. One promising cannabinoid medication for the treatment of MS, Sativex®, which is currently legal in 20 countries, although not yet in the US. Sativex is a mixture of THC and CBD with a 1:1 ratio, and is administered as an oral spray for absorption by the oral mucous membranes, similar to the process of sublingual absorption. The drug is currently making its way through the FDA approval process, and may soon be available in the US.

Researchers Vermersch and Trojano did a study with 281 MS patients who took Sativex® for three months. Patients reported significant improvement in spasticity-related symptoms such as fatigue, pain, spasms, bladder dysfunction, and sleep quality. Patients also reported improved overall quality of life.[47] Numerous other studies on Sativex® have shown similar results. It is not clear which of these therapeutic benefits were due to the presence of THC or CBD, and to what extent.

In a 2015 study done by Italian researchers, only topical CBD was used on mice with an experimental model of MS. The two primary research questions were whether the topical affected the progression of the disease in mice, and whether the topical could reverse paralysis of the legs. The researchers found that "use of the 1% CBD cream improved motor skills, including the reversal of back leg paralysis, a reduction in spinal cord damage, and a decrease in inflammation."[48] While this was a small study done on mice, it provided interesting data that could eventually lead to the introduction of CBD in the treatment of MS.

Further research needs to be done to fully understand the relationship between CBD and MS in humans, but both human and animal trials have shown promise for CBD as a useful method of treatment. Researchers and doctors stress that CBD topical and alternative medicines such as Sativex® are only part of the therapeutic solution for sufferers of MS and similar diseases.

CBD impacts MS via several mechanisms: It decreases the autoimmune inflammatory destruction of the myelin sheath, which slows or stops the progression of the disease. CBD also decreases the symptoms of pain and spasticity. CBD and THC both have positive effects on spasticity, through different mechanisms in the brain and body. CBD also has positive effects on serotonin levels in the brain, improving sleep and depressed mood, both common issues with patients who have MS.

Dosing

Starting adult dose (not recommended in children) 10mg of CBD extract under the tongue, morning, afternoon and bedtime. May increase by 10mg every 4-5 days depending on response to the medication. Once maximum pain relief has been achieved with a certain dose, maintain that dose. Maximum daily dose 200mg. Topical CBD balm can be applied to tight, painful muscle areas three times daily.

Involving Medical Professionals

MS is a serious, and sometimes life-threatening condition. The medications that are prescribed for MS are also serious and need to be managed by a physician. Always involve your neurologist or treating physician with decisions to add CBD or medical cannabis to the treatment of MS.

Chapter 14:
Cancer

As a generalized term, cancer is a disease in which abnormal cells divide uncontrollably and destroy body tissue. These cancerous cells grow abnormally and have the potential to spread and invade other parts of the body. There are over 100 types of cancer that affect humans, with the most common types in industrialized nations being lung, breast, prostate, and colon/rectal cancer.

Cancer does present some general signs and symptoms, but it is important to note that some of these symptoms can be caused by a variety of other conditions, and do not necessarily warrant such a severe diagnosis as cancer. The following are some of the more common cancer symptoms.

Generalized Cancer Symptoms:

- Unexplained weight loss
- Fatigue
- Pain
- Fever
- Skin changes
- Changes in bowel/bladder function
- Non-healing sores
- White patches inside mouth

- Indigestion/trouble swallowing

- Thickening or lump in body

- Nagging cough

Cancer is considered one of the leading causes of death worldwide, with over 12 million cases per year, 7 million of which are ultimately fatal. In the US, it is thought that over 300,000 of the 1.7 million cases of cancer reported annually could be prevented through the adoption of healthier lifestyle choices, such as diet, exercise, and quitting smoking.

The available treatments for cancer are just as variable as the types of cancer. The most common treatments include medication, surgery, chemotherapy, radiation therapy, targeted therapy, immunotherapy, and hormone therapy. Unfortunately, these treatments for cancer can be intensive and may cause some serious side effects.

CBD Treatment

Both CBD and THC impact cancer through several important mechanisms. They increase the death of cancer cells through a mechanism of programmed cell suicide known as apoptosis (a-pop-toe-sis.) All cells have this ability, and frequently undergo the process in response to certain triggers. CBD and THC both trigger a series of intracellular events only in cells that are rapidly dividing (cancer and tumor cells), resulting in apoptosis and cell death. It is not clear in just how many types of cancers this process can occur, but so far, it appears to work in breast, prostate, lung, colon and certain brain cancers.

Angiogenesis is the formation of new blood vessels (arteries and veins.) Cancers promote angiogenesis through various mechanisms to obtain the oxygen and nutrients the cancer needs to grow; thus, a great deal of cancer research has been focused on anti-angiogenesis treatments. A study done by M Solinas et al. examined the relationship between CBD and angiogenesis, with results showing that CBD inhibits angiogenesis via multiple mechanisms. Therefore, the researchers concluded that CBD is a potential effective agent in cancer therapy.[49] Other studies have found similar results in CBD's potential benefit of cancer treatment. Ligresti et al. showed in 2006 that CBD selectively and potently inhibited the growth of different breast tumor cell lines.[50]

Cancers don't merely grow in size; they cause most of their damage by spreading throughout the body and growing new tumors in remote areas of the body. This process is known as metastasis (met-a-stay-sis.) CBD and THC fight cancer by reducing the cancer's ability to migrate, adhere, and invade tissue, resulting in decreased proliferation, and preventing metastasis to other parts of the body.

Not only has CBD shown potential benefits for anti-angiogenesis, but in some studies, it has proven effective at moderating inflammation and reducing the ability of some types of tumor cells to reproduce.[51] Also, as mentioned in previous chapters, CBD has shown benefits with regards to pain management, mood, fatigue, and bowel function, all areas which tend to be negatively impacted by cancer. CBD does not have the effect of improving appetite or reducing nausea, both of which are common problems among chemotherapy patients; rather, the increased appetite and decreased nausea/vomiting associated with cannabis are due to the presence of THC.

Rick Simpson Oil (RSO)

Rick Simpson Oil (RSO), also known as Phoenix Tears (not to be confused with the high-CBD hemp oil sold as Real Scientific Hemp Oil (RSHO™), is a very potent form of thick green/black oil that is very high in THC. It is used at extremely high doses, 1000mg per day, for 60-90 days to treat late-stage cancer. There is not nearly enough hard scientific research to support RSO as a form of cancer treatment, but its benefits have been documented in many case studies and anecdotal reports.

RSO contains highly concentrated amounts of THC, and is very challenging to use without proper education, counseling and guidance. The website www.CureYourOwnCancer.org is a good resource on Rick Simpson Oil, and other alternative treatments for early and late-stage cancer. There are also numerous informational videos on YouTube and elsewhere online about how to use this potentially life-saving oil.

Dosing

While it has shown promise in research studies, there is still not enough official evidence to recommend using CBD in the treatment or prevention of cancer. CBD should have a positive impact on cancer via the mechanisms discussed above, but current data is limited, and a great deal more research still needs to be done to determine the extent of its effects.

At the very least, I can say with confidence that CBD is likely to have a positive therapeutic effect on cancer-related pain, anxiety, depression and mood or sleep disturbance. For more information, please refer to the specific chapter on each of these individual topics.

PART III: MENTAL DISORDERS

Chapter 15:
Depression and Mood

Major Depressive Disorder (MDD), often referred to simply as "depression" or "clinical depression", is a mood disorder defined by chronic feelings of sadness, despondency and dejection. There are many different subtypes of depression, varying in severity, duration, and symptomatology; in general, however, the disease is characterized by a continually low mood and a marked loss of interest in activities to the extent of interfering with or impeding upon one's daily life.

Depression is an extremely common disorder, with over 3 million cases per year in the US alone; in fact, approximately 15% of the adult population is expected to experience at least one depressive episode in their lifetime. While anyone can develop depression at any point in their lives, age and gender seem to play a role in its prevalence, as depression symptoms generally begin to show in adolescence or old age, and four out of five reported cases occur in women.

There is no singular cause or specific contributing factor to the development of depression, but experts have identified a number of diverse individual, societal, and situational factors that seem to contribute, ranging from traumatic events to physical health and even financial circumstances. Researchers also think there is a genetic component to the disease, as depression and related mood disorders often tend to run in families.

Depression Symptoms:

- Irritability

- Persistent sadness

- Fatigue
- Loss of appetite
- Difficulty with sleeping or oversleeping
- Moving slowly
- Thoughts/attempts of suicide
- Aches and pains
- **Types of Depression:**
- Major Depressive Disorder (MDD)
- Persistent Depressive Disorder (PDD)
- Bipolar I Disorder
- Bipolar II Disorder
- Cyclothymic Disorder
- Seasonal Affective Disorder (SAD)
- Psychotic Depression
- Peripartum (Postpartum) Disorder
- Premenstrual Dysphoric Disorder
- Situational Depression (Acute depressive episode)

A temporary feeling of sadness or a generally negative affect does not constitute a psychiatric condition per se, but a long-lasting, chronically low mood, social withdrawal, changes in sleep and appetite, and notable loss of energy or motivation are warning signs that someone may be suffering from a major depressive episode.

Contributing Factors to Depression

Depression is a natural response to loss; It could be the loss of a loved one, a job, a move, trauma, or another difficult life transition resulting in an adverse memory. A period of grieving is a healthy response for navigating through these difficult parts of life, and negative feelings tend to dissipate as the memory fades over time. However, when this sadness lingers or depressive symptoms do not alleviate, it becomes a very serious condition that requires medical attention.

Again, there is no singular, readily identifiable cause of depression, but it is likely affected by both neurobiological and neurochemical components. One widely accepted theory has to do with chemical function and brain structure alteration, as circuits within the brain that regulate moods seem to work less efficiently in depressed individuals. Antidepressant medications are thought to improve communication between brain cells, hence why they have shown to be an effective treatment for some depressed individuals.

The other current treatments available for depression include relaxation and mindfulness techniques, cognitive behavioral therapy (CBT) and psychotherapy. Currently available pharmacological treatments include Selective Serotonin Reuptake Inhibitors (SSRIs), Lithium, valproate, Serotonin–norepinephrine Reuptake Inhibitors (SNRIs), monoamine oxidase inhibitors, tricyclic antidepressant drugs, and partial 5-HT1A receptor agonists. all increase serotonin receptor signaling through either direct or indirect effects.

While antidepressants provide relief for a lot of people, they are ineffective for many others, and do not come without side effects. Addiction, increased suicidal thoughts, loss of sexual desire, weight gain, and anxiety are common side effects of antidepressants.

CBD Treatment

Recently, studies have been done showing that CBD is an alternative treatment for depression, without the psychoactive effects of THC and without the side effects of antidepressants. Another bonus being that relief from CBD occurs within days, whereas antidepressants can take many days or weeks to begin providing relief.

Studies have shown that CBD has a modest affinity for serotonin receptors. It acts as a dose-dependent agonist at the serotonin receptor and can be used to depressive symptomatology.[52] More importantly, CBD works by naturally balancing the cannabinoid tone in the brain and body, resulting in healthier responses to 'adverse memories.' This results in improvement of both anxiety and depression, which often occur at the same time. Long-term daily use of CBD extract can have therapeutic effects on preventing and decreasing the symptoms of depression and lifting a person's mood.

A recent study in rodents suggests that CBD can provide novel and rapid and sustained antidepressant effects.[53] These effects may be related to rapid changes in synaptic plasticity in the medial pre-frontal cortex (mPFC) through activation of the BDNF-TrkB signaling pathway.

In a study done by Shoval G, et al. adult male rats (with the equivalent of human depression) were given CBD orally or were in a placebo group. Different tests were used with the rats to determine the effect of CBD.[54] The results showed that CBD had a prohedonic effect on the rats treated; in a novel object exploration test and a locomotion test, CBD treated rats showed increased exploration and locomotion. The findings of this study express the beneficial effects CBD may have for the treatment of depression.

As will be discussed in a later chapter on anxiety and stress, the hippocampus is one of the centers in the brain that has to do with memory storage and processing. The hippocampus has very high levels of cannabinoid receptors. Like several other centers in the brain, the hippocampus has an abundance of CB1 receptors. However, recent research has shown that there are also many CB2 receptors in the hippocampus.

The new research shows that stimulation of these CB2 receptors raises the excitation threshold. What this means in practice is that increased CB2 stimulation with CBD or some other cannabinoid medications decreases the hippocampus' response to stored adverse memories. Since chronic sadness and depression are often due to a sense of 'loss' associated with an adverse memory, this results in decreased symptoms of depression and an improved mood.

Depression and THC

Depression can be a side-effect of excessive cannabis use, especially in younger users. This is due to the impact on the hippocampus and amygdala (emotional center in the brain) from high levels of THC. These side effects almost always occur with recreational use of cannabis. Too much and too frequent use of THC, usually observed in serious recreational users, can cause a depressed mood.

Medical-grade cannabis are those strains used to treat medical conditions. Medical-grade cannabis has a ratio of CBD to THC of 1:1 or higher, which means there are equal or greater amounts of CBD in the cannabis, compared to the amounts of THC. For example, the cannabis strains to treat seizures contain a 20:1 ratio of CBD to THC, or twenty times more CBD than THC. This ratio is 1:1 in Sativex® and most other strains used for medical conditions. Because the effects of CBD counter those of THC, adverse reactions are not likely to occur in these balanced 1:1 medications, so they are not associated with depression.

CBD Extract

Starting adult dose (not recommended in children) 10mg of CBD extract under the tongue, morning, afternoon and bedtime. May increase by 10mg every 4-5 days depending on response to the medication. Once maximum symptom relief has been achieved with a certain dose, maintain that dose. Maximum daily dose 200mg.

As I have mentioned before, CBD can be beneficial for mood regulation and preventing the development of depressive symptoms; however, treatment of acute or sudden onset of severe depression or suicidal thoughts with CBD is not well-studied. These cases should be considered as medical emergencies, requiring immediate medical attention. Other FDA-approved antidepressant medications, readily available through your doctor, are likely to be much more beneficial and have more rapid onset in these circumstances.

Treatment doesn't always work

Medicine is an art, more than it is a science. Sometimes the recommended treatment doesn't work. It may not work because the dose wasn't correct, or it may not work because the underlying condition causing the symptoms are more severe than originally thought.

Start out with extract. If the maximum doses of CBD are not getting you enough symptom relief, it is time to go back to your physician for some advice.

Involving Medical Professionals

Depression is a serious, and sometimes even life-threatening, psychiatric condition. The medications used for treatment of depression need to be managed by a physician. Always involve your psychiatrist or treating physician with decisions to add CBD or medical cannabis to the treatment of these conditions

Chapter 16:
Insomnia

A sleep disorder is defined as "changes in sleep habits or patterns that negatively affect a person's health or function." There are many types of sleep disorders, with insomnia being the most prevalent, followed by sleep apnea. Insomnia is a disorder in which people have difficulty falling and/or staying asleep; primary insomnia and secondary insomnia are the two main types of the disorder. Primary insomnia is when a person has sleep problems that are not correlated or caused by another problem or health condition; secondary insomnia, on the other hand, is caused by something else, such as depression, arthritis, cancer pain, or substance abuse.

Insomnia Symptoms:

- Difficulty falling asleep
- Waking up often during the night
- Having trouble going back to sleep
- Waking up too early in the morning
- Feeling tired upon waking
- Irritability
- Memory/concentration problems

It is thought that as many as 1 in 4 people suffer from some form of insomnia, and that most people will experience insomnia during their lifetime.[55] For a health care provider to diagnose insomnia, they might do a few different things. A physical exam, a medical and sleep history, and possibly keeping a sleep diary for a week will help a healthcare provider better understand the nature of one's insomnia. Sometimes people are referred to a sleep center, where they undergo a sleep study, either in a lab or with a machine at home.

There are many treatment options to aid in improving insomnia symptoms. Adjusting sleep habits, such as improving one's sleep hygiene, undergoing light therapy, and cognitive behavioral therapy are all non-medicated options to improve insomnia symptoms. Another common treatment for insomnia is medication such as sleeping pills, but these can come with unpleasant and even dangerous side effects. Many sleep aids are addictive and can greatly increase the likelihood of an unexpected overdose of opioids among those taking opioids for pain. It is for these reasons that most sleeping pills are not recommended for long-term or daily use.

CBD Treatment

While there isn't a great deal of clinically proven evidence for the use of CBD to treat insomnia, a few studies have indicated that it has potential benefits, but not in the way one might think. Unlike THC, CBD has been found to be mildly energizing at moderate doses, rather than having a sedative effect. At much higher doses, however, it can be sedating. Numerous studies have been done with high-THC cannabis that have found cannabis as an effective treatment for insomnia. CBD, on the other hand, can still be effective in aiding in the treatment of insomnia, but in a different way than THC cannabis.

In a study done by Nicholas et al., 15mg of THC proved to be sedative, while 15mg of CBD had the effect of increasing alertness as well as increasing wake activity during sleep and counteracting the sedative effect of the THC.[56] This study, as well as a few others, found that CBD caused humans or rodents to be alert rather than sleepy. Therefore, it has been concluded that while CBD isn't an effective treatment for sleep disorders in terms of falling and staying asleep, it is effective in reducing sleepiness and fatigue. A common symptom of people with sleep disorders is feeling tired throughout the day as the result of too little sleep, or unfulfilling sleep; CBD can aid in treating this symptom by providing increased alertness and energy throughout the day.

On a separate note, CBD has been shown to significantly reduce anxiety and feelings of stress (this is discussed in detail in the next chapter.) By helping to reduce feelings of anxiety and helping to calm the spiraling thoughts and rumination that tend to be attributed to onset insomnia, CBD may yet prove to be a beneficial component of a successful insomnia treatment program.

Dosing

Because CBD near bedtime can actually increase wakefulness, dosing around this time is not recommended for individuals with insomnia. However, if perceived stress or anxious feelings are causing one to have difficulty falling asleep, consider a trial of CBD around an hour before bedtime. I will discuss at length how CBD may be useful for anxiety relief in the next chapter.

Chapter 17:
Anxiety, PTSD, and Stress

Generalized Anxiety Disorder (GAD), more simply known as "anxiety," is a mental health disorder that is characterized by feelings of worry, fear, nervousness, or unease.[57] These mental symptoms are often associated with physical symptoms, such as rapid pulse, shallow rapid breathing, and dry mouth. These feelings are strong enough that they interfere with a person's daily life and activities. It is considered a common disorder, with over 3 million cases a year just in the US. "Anxiety" is considered a general term that includes different conditions, including panic, social anxiety and various phobias. In addition to GAD, in this chapter we will discuss Post-Traumatic Stress Disorder (PTSD) and perceived "stress.

Stress is a major risk factor for the development of mood and anxiety disorders; novel approaches to using CBD to mitigate the deleterious effects of stress could have broad clinical applications. Animal studies have suggested that stress inhibits overall endocannabinoid functioning, so pharmacological augmentation of ECS by CBD may be a viable strategy to treat mood and anxiety disorders.[58] In addition, the presence of the ECS in stress-responsive neural circuits suggests that it may play a critical role in regulating neuroendocrine and behavioral responses to stress.

There are ECS receptors in about a dozen centers of the brain that relate to various aspects of emotional response and adverse memory extinction.[57] Because of this, CBD has been postulated to have several novel therapeutic effects on anxiety, depression, PTSD, OCD, and phobias, as well as psychosis and schizophrenia.

Generalized Anxiety Disorder (GAD) Symptoms:

- Panic

- Fear
- Unease
- Shortness of breath
- Dry mouth
- Sleep problems
- Inability to stay calm or still
- Tense muscles
- Dizziness
- Post-traumatic Stress Disorder (PTSD) Symptoms:
- Nightmares
- Flashbacks
- Avoidance of triggering situations (situations that bring back traumatic memories)
- Heightened reactivity to stimuli
- Anxiety
- Depressed mood

While researchers have yet to pinpoint a specific cause or trigger for anxiety disorders, several factors play a role. Environmental stress, changes in the brain, and genetics can all be contributing factors. Anxiety disorders, like many other mental disorders, tend to run in families. There are no specific lab tests that can diagnose an anxiety disorder, but a medical doctor will ask questions about medical history, symptoms, and may do some tests to rule out other medical conditions. A doctor may then suggest a psychologist, psychiatrist, or mental health professional; these mental health specialists will ask questions and use tools and tests to find out more about the anxiety.

One thing these conditions have in common is that they are all in response to 'adverse memories.' We store scenes of trauma differently than other types of memories, imprinting them in the hippocampus center in our brain. For most people, these adverse memories gradually fade over time; However, some recall their traumatic memories much more vividly and actively, especially if the traumatic incident occurs at a very young age or is of a particularly disturbing nature.

When these adverse memories don't fade right away, the constant, nagging memory of the traumatic incident (and corresponding fear that the incident will recur) causes the release of adrenaline. Adrenaline, known colloquially as the 'fight or flight' hormone, was developed evolutionarily to protect our ancestors from attacks by predators or other dangerous situations, e.g. a sabertooth tiger attack. Once adrenaline is released into our body, blood rushes to our muscles to prepare us to either run away from danger or fight. This results in rapid heartbeat, rapid shallow breaths, dry mouth, trembling hands and often a feeling of impending doom. This is known physiologically as the "stress response," and works through a complex system that connects the emotional part of the brain to the body through the Hypothalamic-Pituitary-Adrenal (HPA) axis.

In the modern world, we may not encounter such forms of acute danger as frequently as our primitive ancestors did, but our adrenal glands still tend to remain constantly stimulated at lower levels in response to the many perceived threats and general stressors of modern-day society. When this constant, perceived threat doesn't resolve itself over time, these long-term, low-level feelings of chronic stress and anxiety cause the excessive release of our body's steroid hormone, cortisol, which is associated with elevated blood pressure, increased storage of fat, and reduced immune response. This wearing down of the adrenal glands over time in turn causes a condition known as adrenal fatigue. The feeling of being stressed out or suffering from chronic stress is not a diagnosable mental disorder per se, but mental health specialists do recognize that chronic stress can lead to adrenal fatigue and 'burnout.'

Treating anxiety disorders differs from person to person depending on their symptoms, medical history, and severity of the disorder. For some people self-care treatments such as: physical exercise, stress management, relaxation, avoiding alcohol, lessening caffeine, and having a healthy diet, are enough to treat the anxiety disorder so no further treatment is needed; for others, medications like antidepressants, anxiolytics, or sedatives are used to lessen the symptoms of anxiety. Cognitive behavioral therapy, psychotherapy, and meditation have also proven to be helpful in many individuals with anxiety disorders. [59]

Anxiety

Anxiety is a very common symptom, and part of a spectrum of psychological conditions that include generalized anxiety disorder (GAD), social anxiety disorder (SAD), panic disorder, PTSD and Obsessive-Compulsive Disorder (OCD). Anxiety is associated with a plethora of somatic complaints and rumination. It is an unpleasant feeling of worry, uneasiness, or dread over anticipated events or a response to a perceived threat. There are many diagnoses that include anxiety as part of the syndrome, including PTSD, OCD and phobias.

The current treatments available for anxiety include relaxation and mindfulness techniques, yoga, cognitive behavioral therapy (CBT) and psychotherapy. Current clinically utilized pharmacological treatments for affective disorders are primarily based on augmenting monoamines stimulation in the brain. Currently available pharmacological treatments include serotonin reuptake inhibitors, serotonin–norepinephrine reuptake inhibitors, benzodiazepines, monoamine oxidase inhibitors, tricyclic antidepressant drugs, and partial 5-HT1A receptor agonists. Anxiety disorder is often poorly controlled by the currently available drugs, and only about 30% of the subjects achieve true recovery or remission without residual symptomatology.[59]

During repeated exposure to aversive stimuli, the ECS upregulates in limbic structures, resulting in dampened neural activity in stress circuits, which could contribute to stress habituation. CNS endocannabinoids levels predict acute stress-induced anxiety, and reversal of stress-induced endocannabinoid deficiency is a key therapy for anxiety. Studies have shown that CBD can be used to treat acute anxiety-related or panic symptoms, and for ongoing treatment for multiple anxiety disorders.[60]

Animal models and several human trials have shown that CBD can be helpful for reducing anxiety in various clinical scenarios and conditions. Studies involving animal models, performing a variety of experiments such as the forced swimming test (FST), elevated plus maze (EPM) and Vogel conflict test (VCT), suggest that CBD exhibited both anti-anxiety and antidepressant effects via serotonin and ECS mechanisms.[61]

CBD has anxiety-reducing action via CB1, TRPV1 and 5-HT1A receptors. There is also accumulating evidence from animal studies investigating the effects of cannabidiol on fear memory processing, indicating that it reduces learned fear, which is relevant to phobias and PTSD. CBD does so by reducing fear expression acutely, and by disrupting fear memory reconsolidation and enhancing fear extinction, both of which can result in a lasting reduction of learned fear.

PTSD

Various phobias and post-traumatic stress disorder (PTSD) are characterized by abnormal and persistent memories of fear-related contexts and cues. The effects of psychological treatments such as exposure therapy are often only temporary, and many of the available medications can be ineffective and have adverse side effects.

Mounting evidence indicates that CBD reduces learned fear in different ways. CBD decreases fear expression acutely; CBD disrupts memory reconsolidation, leading to sustained fear attenuation upon memory retrieval; finally, CBD enhances extinction, the psychological process by which exposure therapy inhibits learned fear; and 4: Auditory fear expression is also reduced acutely by CBD.

Phobias

Phobias are postulated to operate through similar learned fear. These conditions respond to treatment that improves disrupted memory reconsolidation with associated sustained fear attenuation upon memory retrieval, and poor adverse memory extinction. CBD, therefore, is postulated to improve both acute and chronic phobias.

CBD Treatment

The hippocampus is one of the centers in the brain pertaining to memory storage and memory processing. The hippocampus is also intimately involved with regulating the HPA axis discussed above. The hippocampus has very high levels of cannabinoid receptors. Like several other centers in the brain, the hippocampus has an abundance of CB1 receptors; however, recent research has shown that there are also many CB2 receptors in the hippocampus. The new research shows that stimulation of these CB2 receptors raises the excitation threshold. What this means in practice is that increased CB2 stimulation with CBD or other cannabinoid medications decreases the responsiveness of the hippocampus to stored adverse memories. Because anxiety, perceived stress, and PTSD are all caused by 'fear' of the recurrence of adverse memory, this increase in CB2 stimulation results in decreased symptoms of such conditions.

In a study done by researchers in Brazil, it was found that CBD helped in treating anxiety disorders.[60] They reviewed studies that used animal models, healthy volunteers, and people suffering from anxiety to conduct their research. In one particular study using mice, researchers investigated fear-induced behaviors caused by a snake in a maze. They found that the mice that were pre-treated with CBD had significant reductions in defensive immobility and explosive flight, as compared to the non-treated control group. Even with these reductions, the mice treated with CBD showed no alteration in risk assessment and defensive attention. The results of this study provide evidence that CBD could be effective in the aid of panic attacks.

In the same review, the researchers found similar findings in human studies with CBD. Researchers conducted a study with the intent to investigate CBD and anxiolytic interaction using a group of healthy volunteers. The volunteers were asked to speak in front of a video camera for a few minutes, as public speaking is an anxiety trigger for many. CBD, as well as diazepam and ipsapirone, was shown to significantly lessen anxiety associated with public speaking. The conclusion of this review of studies involving CBD is as follows:

"Together, the results from laboratory animals, healthy volunteers, and patients with anxiety disorders support the proposition of CBD as a new drug with anxiolytic properties. Because it has no psychoactive effects and does not affect cognition; has an adequate safety profile, good tolerability, positive results in trials with humans, and a broad-spectrum of pharmacological actions, CBD appears to be the cannabinoid compound that is closer to have its preliminary findings in anxiety translated into clinical practice."

Another study regarding CBD and anxiety focused on functional neuroimaging rather than self-assessment scales and physiological measures. In this study, patients with social anxiety disorder (SAD), were given either 200mg of oral CBD or a placebo. Relative to the patients given a placebo, those given CBD showed significantly decreased anxiety and changes in the brain in association with lower anxiety. The researchers concluded that their results suggest that "CBD reduces anxiety in SAD" and that this is "related to its effect on activity in the limbic and paralimbic brain areas."

Hampson has shown that the anxiety-relieving effect of CBD can be blocked by a serotonin antagonist, indicating that this receptor is in part responsible for mediating the anxiolytic effects of CBD. Curiously, Hampson's current data suggests that in addition to binding directly to serotonin receptors, CBD may also act by altering the functionality of this receptor in such a way as to enhance its binding efficiency. In other words, CBD may actually magnify the effect of serotonin, in addition to directly activating the serotonin receptor.

Panic and THC

Panic, agitation and anxiety are all side effects that can occur with some regularity in people who use cannabis. These side effects are due to the impact on the hippocampus and amygdala (emotional center in the brain) from high levels of THC. These side effects almost always occur with recreational use of cannabis. Too much THC, such as 20-30mg in a short period of time, (especially in strains containing low levels of CBD to mitigate the effects of THC), often results in these unpleasant symptoms. These symptoms can be treated with 20-60mg of CBD oil administered sublingually (under the tongue.)

"Medical-grade cannabis" refers to strains specifically designed to treat medical conditions. Medical-grade cannabis has a ratio of CBD to THC of 1:1 or higher, meaning it contains an equal or greater amount of CBD as compared to the amount of THC. For example, the cannabis strains to treat seizures are 20:1, with twenty times more CBD than THC. The ratio of CBD to THC in strains used for most other medical conditions, as well as Sativex® spray, is 1:1, containing equal amounts of CBD and THC. These balanced medications, in regular doses, are not associated with anxiety, panic or agitation.

CBD Extract:

The recommended starting dose of CBD for adults (not recommended in children) is ~10mg of extract under the tongue, morning, afternoon and bedtime. This dose may be increased by 10mg every 4-5 days, depending on the individual's response to the medication. Once maximum symptom relief has been achieved with a certain dose, that dose should be maintained, with a maximum daily dose not exceeding 200mg.

Long-term daily use of CBD extract can have therapeutic effects on preventing and decreasing the symptoms of anxiety, PTSD, and other panic-related conditions. As opposed to the long-term varieties of these conditions, treatment of acute or sudden-onset cases of anxiety, PTSD, panic and phobias with CBD is not well-studied. Pharmaceutical medications for these conditions offer much more rapid onset of symptom relief and are readily available by prescription from your doctor. For sudden onset of symptoms, an adult dose (not recommended in children) is 20-60mg extract under the tongue, one time daily.

When treating any condition with CBD, it is recommended that you start out with CBD extract. If the maximum dose of CBD is not getting you enough symptom relief, it is time to go back to your physician and reassess your treatment plan.

Treatment doesn't always work

Contrary to common wisdom, effective medicine is truly an art more than it is a science. I say this because medical care is best administered on an individual, case-by-case basis; there is no "one size fits all" treatment for most conditions, and a certain degree of trial and error may be involved before a patient gets the treatment they actually need. For any number of reasons, sometimes the textbook recommended treatment doesn't work; this may be because the medication wasn't dosed properly, or perhaps because the underlying condition causing the symptoms is more severe than originally thought. It is important to work closely and collaboratively with your doctor and express your own personal concerns about your condition in order to find the treatment that is right for you.

Involving Medical Professionals

Generalized anxiety and chronic stress symptoms can be very serious, and sometimes represent deep and debilitating psychiatric conditions. Medications for anxiety and stress-related symptoms need to be carefully and attentively regulated by a qualified physician. Always involve your psychiatrist or treating physician with your decision to add CBD or medical cannabis to the treatment of these conditions.

Chapter 18:
Obsessive-Compulsive Disorder

Obsessive-Compulsive Disorder (OCD) is a chronic anxiety disorder, characterized by intrusive and nagging thoughts (obsessions) that lead to reflexive and repetitive behaviors (compulsions). Obsessions are repeated urges, thoughts, or mental images that cause discomfort or anxiety. Compulsions are repetitive behaviors that a person with OCD feels the urge to do in response to obsessive thought. Because these behaviors are compulsive, there is no decision-making involved, and the person suffering from OCD may not even be aware that they are exhibiting compulsive behavior.

Approximately 3.3 million Americans are afflicted with OCD; onset usually begins during puberty or in one's late teens. In most cases of OCD, it represents a minor annoyance to the OCD sufferer; in other cases, it can cause extreme distress, evolving into a debilitating condition that effectively inhibits people from going about their normal daily life.

An OCD individual usually experiences obsession over a particular thought or phobia. For example, if an individual has germophobia, the resulting compulsion would be a nagging urge to excessively clean or wash one's hands. In other cases, OCD can manifest as a tic disorder, resulting in automatic bodily movements or vocal tics. The compulsive behavior may be technically unnecessary or even irrational, but anxiety over what will happen if they don't fulfill these compulsive urges generally makes the OCD individual feel helpless and unable to avoid either their obsessive thoughts or the action that follows.

While its exact causes are unknown, there are several common risk factors associated with OCD. Genetics, brain structure and functioning, and environmental factors all play a role in the likelihood of a person developing OCD. For example, as is the case with many mental disorders, people who experience abuse or trauma in childhood may adopt deviant or pathological behaviors as coping mechanisms, and therefore, are at an increased risk for developing conditions such as OCD later on.

Diagnosis

While some people with OCD do notice their obsessive thoughts and are aware of its effect on their functioning, in most cases, particularly in children, the person does not realize their behavior is out of the ordinary. With cases of OCD in children, it is often parents or teachers who initially take notice of the compulsive behavior(s) and bring them to the attention of a healthcare provider. The signs and symptoms of this condition might be noticeable to the OCD sufferer and others, but only a licensed mental health professional can actually diagnose OCD.

Obsession Symptoms:

- Repeated unwanted ideas
- Aggressive impulses
- Fear of contamination
- Images of hurting someone
- Intense need to keep things symmetrical or in perfect order
- Compulsion Symptoms:
- Excessive cleaning/hand washing
- Constant checking
- Constant counting
- Repeated counting

- Repeated cleaning
- Arranging items to face certain way

While the points above represent some of the most common thoughts and behaviors associated with OCD, these symptoms vary widely from individual to individual, so they should be considered by no means an exhaustive list.

Treatment of OCD generally involves some combination of antidepressants and/or anxiolytic (anti-anxiety) medications and psychotherapy. So far, antidepressant medications, specifically Selective Serotonin Reuptake Inhibitors (SSRIs), seem to be the most effective.

CBD Treatment

These conditions respond to treatment that improves disrupted memory reconsolidation with associated sustained fear attenuation upon memory retrieval, and poor adverse memory extinction. CBD, therefore, is postulated to improve both acute and chronic symptoms of OCD. While antidepressants do provide relief for a great number of people, they do not come without side effects. Increased suicidal thoughts, loss of libido, weight gain, and anxiety are all common side effects of SSRI antidepressants.

Recent studies have demonstrated that CBD can be an effective alternative treatment for OCD, without the psychoactive effects of THC and without the side effects of antidepressants. Another benefit of CBD is that symptom relief begins within a few days, whereas antidepressants can take weeks or months before there is any noticeable effect. More importantly, CBD works by naturally balancing the endocannabinoid tone in the brain and body, resulting in increased neuroplasticity (i.e. the brain's natural ability to adapt to and mitigate negative thoughts or feelings and adverse memories.) This structural change is permanent, resulting in effective, long-term symptom relief, even after the use of CBD is discontinued.

There has not been a great deal of human research on the use of cannabinoid medications (THC and CBD) specifically for the treatment of OCD. However, based on what we know about how CBD works in the brain, it is likely that CBD decreases the brain's fear response to the recall of an adverse memory.

This is how it helps people with anxiety, depression, and OCD; By decreasing the level of 'fear' associated with not doing the compulsive behavior, the compulsion becomes less intense and more manageable. It is possible that CBD may decrease the prevalence of obsessive thoughts as well.

Recent research has shown support for the role CBD could play in treating OCD. A study by a team of Brazilian researchers, first published in October of 2013 in the journal Fundamental & Clinical Pharmacology, investigated the effects of CBD on rats. The rats were first administered a chemical that leads to hormonal, physiological and behavioral effects, and is known to induce panic attacks, as well as to worsen OCD symptoms. Later, the rats were given CBD, and were re-evaluated with regard to obsessive-compulsive activity; the rats were shown to be significantly calmer and less prone to anxious behaviors once the CBD had taken effect.[62]

Based on the results of their study, the researchers determined that CBD delivers notable anti-compulsive effects, likely due to the interaction between the serotonergic and endocannabinoid system. Because CBD does not come with any severe side effects, it should be considered as a potential alternative for OCD patients who may be experiencing negative effects from their current medications (such as antidepressants) and are seeking other treatment options.

Dosing

The same dosing rules apply to the treatment of OCD with CBD as with all other physical and mental disorders mentioned in this book.

Involving Medical Professionals

OCD can be a serious psychiatric condition that can affect someone's social life and work. The medications for OCD need to be managed by a physician. Always involve your psychiatrist or treating physician with decisions to add CBD or medical cannabis to the treatment of these conditions.

Chapter 19:
Autism Spectrum Disorder

An absence of empirical data appears to have resulted in a growing body of anecdotal evidence espousing the benefits of CBD for children with autism spectrum disorder (ASD.) A 2018 review of the scientific literature for CBD and ASD found no research or even case reported published on the topic.[63] The authors concluded, “there is a paucity of literature supporting the clinical evidence for use of CBD in ASD. CBD and similar products remain a promising yet unproven intervention in the treatment of children with ASD.”

Autism Spectrum Disorder (ASD), commonly known as autism, is a serious developmental disorder that impairs the ability to communicate and interact. The disorder varies greatly in severity and characteristics, creating a “spectrum” of skills, symptoms, and levels of disability. ASD is considered a somewhat common disorder, with over 200,000 cases a year. While females are affected by ASD, it is more common in males and is usually diagnosed during young childhood years. Seizure disorder occurs in about one third of the cases. It is felt that abnormalities can cause changes in brain activity disrupting the nerve cells in certain centers in the brain.

Until recently there was another condition called Asperger’s syndrome, which was separate from Autism Disorder. However, in the latest edition of the Diagnostic and Statistical Manual of Mental Disorders (DSM-5), there are no longer subcategories within the label of Autism Spectrum Disorder, which includes a range of characteristics and severity within one category.

Signs of autism tend to appear early in development; a child can be reliably diagnosed with ASD by the age of two. A doctor will look a child’s behavior and development, as well as discuss the child’s behavior with a parent. Diagnosing ASD in adults is not as simple as with young children, and the testing for adults is still being refined. Adults who may suspect ASD can speak with a psychologist or psychiatrist with ASD expertise about signs and symptoms.

While scientists and doctors still don't know the exact cause of ASD, several risk factors have been identified. According to NIMH, these may include:

Gender—boys are more likely to be diagnosed with ASD than girls

Having a sibling with ASD

Having older parents (a mother who was 35 or older, and/or a father who was 40 or older when the baby was born)

Genetics—about 20% of children with ASD also have certain genetic conditions. Those conditions include Down syndrome, fragile X syndrome, and tuberous sclerosis, among others.

In recent years, the number of children diagnosed with ASD has increased. Experts disagree about whether this shows a true increase in ASD, since the diagnostic criteria has changed in recent years as well. Also, many more parents and doctors now know about the disorder, so parents are more likely to have their children screened, and more doctors are able to properly diagnose ASD, even in adulthood.

There is currently no cure for ASD, but a number of therapies and treatments exist. Early treatment for ASD is crucial as it can help an individual learn new skills, make the most of their strengths, and reduce certain difficulties. In some early interventions, therapists will use highly structured and intensive training sessions to aid children in developing positive social and language skills, while discouraging negative behaviors. It has also been shown to be helpful if the family of the child with ASD participates in therapy, to help them cope with the challenges of living with someone with ASD.

Medication is another treatment option for ASD, but it does not cure or even necessarily treat the main symptoms. It can help with seizures and symptoms like obsessive-compulsive disorder (OCD), depression, anxiety or severe behavioral problems. But as with many medications, sometimes the side effects of the medication are worse than the symptoms themselves.

Behavioral Symptoms:

- Inappropriate social interaction
- Compulsive behavior
- Persistent repetition of words
- Impulsivity
- Poor eye contact
- Self-harm
- Repetitive movements
- Cognitive Symptoms
- Problems paying attention
- Intense interest in limited number of things
- Developmental Symptoms
- Speech delay in children
- Learning disability
- Psychological Symptoms:
- Depression
- Anxiety
- Lack of awareness of others' emotions

- Other Symptoms:
- Tics
- Sensitivity to lights, sounds, touch, and smells
- Change in voice
- Early indicators of ASD may include:
- No babbling or pointing by age 1
- No response to name
- Poor eye contact
- No single words by age 16 months
- No two-word phrases by age 2
- Excessive lining up of toys or objects
- No smiling or social responsiveness
- Later indicators of ASD may include:
- Impaired ability to make friends or initiate/sustain conversations with others
- Repetitive or unusual use of language
- Inflexible adherence to specific rituals or routines
- Repetitive or unusual use of language
- Absence/impairment of social or imaginative play

CBD and ASD

Considering that the symptoms and severity of ASD varies among individuals, treatment options are varied as well. Cannabis, particularly CBD or a combination of THC and CBD with high CBD and low THC, have been found to be effective treatments. These high CBD/low THC medications are also effective for the treatment of childhood epilepsy. CBD is also known for having both analgesic (pain reducing) and anxiolytic (anti-anxiety) effects, effectively treating many of the symptoms of ASD.

In a study done by the University of California, the researchers found that "CBD regulates emotion and focus, acting as a neuroprotective against further nerve cell damage. In the autistic patient, mood can be regulated with oral doses of cannabis… CBD has reduced anxiety, rage and hostility in patients by inducing a relaxed, steady and calm demeanor. When including the positive effect of cannabis on seizures, the potential use of CBD for treatment of ASD because very real."[63]

Dr. Adi Aran, an Israeli doctor, is currently conducting a first of its kind clinical trial involving CBD for treating autism in children and young adults. Aran was experiencing parent's asking for cannabis for their children with ASD and feeling uncomfortable prescribing something he hadn't researched, Aran conducted an observational study on 70 of his autistic patients.[64]

The results demonstrated that CBD provided significant improvements in many of the children. Some children no longer threw tantrums or hurt themselves, while others were more communicative. It is the positive results of this observational study that has led to him conducting his two-year clinical trial.

Dosing

For those ASD patients with epilepsy, the dosing guidelines found in the seizure and epilepsy chapter should be followed. In general, CBD has been shown to be helpful for long term control of the number and severity of the seizures. Because of this, use a whole-plant extract that is swished inside of the front of the mouth.

The starting dose is for children is ½ milligram per pound/weight, divided into three, equal, daily doses (morning, afternoon, and bedtime.) So, a child weighing 100lbs would take approximately 17mg, three times a day, for a total of 50mg.) This dose can be doubled after four days to see if there is further improvement.

Continue to increase by ½ milligram per pound, every four days; the second dose for a child weighing 100 lbs would be 1mg per lb or 100mg, divided into three doses of 33mg each. Keep increasing dose gradually until improvement plateaus.

The maximum recommended dose for children is 5mg per pound, per day. THC, sometimes present in "High-CBD" products, can actually aggravate epilepsy, so be sure the products you choose are certified laboratory tested with low amounts of THC (less than 0.3%).

For treatment of patients with ASD without epilepsy, the most important symptoms are those of decreased social interaction, poor mood, anxiety and tantrums. CBD is safely started at ½ milligram per pound/weight, divided into three equal daily doses (morning, afternoon, and bedtime.) So, a child weighing 100lbs would take approximately 17mg, three times a day, for a total of 50mg.

This dose can be doubled after four days to see if there is further improvement. Continue to increase by ½ milligram per pound, every four days. The second dose for a 100lb child would be 1mg per lb or 100mg, divided into three doses of 33mg each. Keep increasing until improvement plateaus. The maximum recommended dose is 5mg per pound a day.

Involving Medical Professionals

Childhood and adult-onset epilepsy both represent a significant and potentially life-threatening condition. Although it has not been reported, it is possible that the large doses of CBD required to control seizures may change the liver enzymes' metabolism of many prescription drugs used to treat epilepsy.

Because of the complexity and severity of seizure disorder, and possibility medication interaction with CBD or medical marijuana, patients and guardians of patients with epilepsy should always work closely with their neurologist to determine if adding CBD or medical marijuana is appropriate. Neurologists usually have little or no training on the subject, and often won't actually recommend the CBD to a patient with epilepsy; However, then may give their permission to add CBD to the patient's treatment plan.

Chapter 20: Psychosis and Schizophrenia

Psychosis and schizophrenia are two intense mental disorders that result in greatly disturbed thoughts, moods, and behaviors. There are many different forms of psychosis, some where the symptoms last only a few hours, and sometimes the psychosis lasts a lifetime. Schizophrenia is an inherited condition, marked by the onset of psychosis in young adulthood.

Psychosis Symptoms:

- Depression
- Difficulty concentrating
- Suspiciousness
- Delusions
- Disorganized speech
- Withdrawal from loved ones
- Sleep troubles
- Anxiety
- Suicidal thoughts
- Schizophrenia Symptoms:

- Thoughts/experiences that seem out of touch with reality
- Disorganized speech or behavior
- Decreased participating in daily activities
- Memory/concentration difficulties

With both conditions, symptoms vary greatly from person to person. Psychosis is characterized by thoughts and emotions that are so impaired it causes a disconnection from reality. Delusions, defined as "idiosyncratic beliefs or impressions that are firmly maintained despite being contradicted by what is generally accepted as reality or rational argument, typically a symptom of a mental disorder," are a common symptom of psychosis; Hallucinations, meanwhile, are "experiences involving the apparent perception of something not present," and are also telltale signs of psychosis or a psychotic episode. These sudden-onset indicators of psychosis can be frightening for the person experiencing these thoughts, potentially causing them to hurt themselves or others.

The causes and risk factors of psychosis are not completely known, but there are many theories. For example, certain illnesses that attack the brain, such as Alzheimer's, Parkinson's, brain tumors, dementia, strokes, or HIV have been shown to cause psychosis in some people. Other risk factors might include genetics, a family member with psychosis, or children born with a certain genetic mutation. Some types of psychosis can be brought on by specific circumstances, such as drug and alcohol abuse; brief psychotic episodes, for example, can be brought on by extreme personal stress.

The most common theory is that psychotic symptoms may be due to inflammation in certain centers of the brain. If this is true, then the ECS can have an important role in mediating the inflammation. However, research is early and tenuous at this time.

CBD Treatment

Treatments for schizophrenia and chronic psychosis can be as varied as the different types and symptoms. Some of the currently available interventions include medication, psychotherapy, hospital or residential programs, brain stimulation, or substance abuse treatment. These treatments have been shown to be successful in many cases, but some of them, such as certain medications, have severe side effects.

CBD is a potential treatment option for certain types of psychosis. In numerous studies, CBD has been found to inhibit the episodic psychotic-like symptoms sometimes induced by THC. It has been shown to have antipsychotic effects, which is part of the reason it has potential as treatment or psychiatric conditions. In an online study done of over 1800 subjects, cannabis with a high CBD content was "associated with significantly lower degrees of psychotic symptoms, providing further support of the antipsychotic potential of cannabidiol". [65, 66]

In another study done specifically in relation to schizophrenia, the researchers concluded: "The anti-inflammatory and immunomodulatory effects of the non-intoxicating phytocannabinoid [CBD] are well established. Preliminary data reviewed in this paper suggest that CBD in combinations with a CB1 receptor neutral antagonist could not only augment the effects of antipsychotic drugs but also target the metabolic, inflammatory and stress-related components of the schizophrenia phenotype."[67]

Many other studies have found similar results. What these studies and research portray is that CBD definitely has antipsychotic effects that could be useful in treating psychiatric conditions; however, as with many of the conditions for which CBD treatment has shown promise, more research and clinical studies need to be done to find out more information and potential treatment plans.

Psychosis and THC

A temporary episode of psychosis can be a scary side effect in people who use cannabis, especially with higher doses of THC and in younger users. These side effects almost always occur with recreational users of cannabis. Too much and too frequent use of THC in younger persons, especially if there is a family history or prior history of psychosis or schizophrenia. Still, there has been an ongoing and unresolved debate regarding THC causing schizophrenia, and available research is limited.

A review of the available evidence would suggest that recreational use of THC can uncover a person's predisposition for eventually getting schizophrenia; that is, a person who was already genetically at risk for eventually developing schizophrenia and started consuming the high amounts of THC seen in recreational use, would experience earlier onset of schizophrenia symptoms than they would had they not used THC.[68] People with a prior history of acute psychotic episodes are at greatly increased risk for recurrent psychotic episodes with the use of THC, especially large recreational amounts of THC.

However, this is not the case with 'medical-grade' cannabis, or those particular strains used to treat medical conditions. Medical-grade cannabis has a ratio of CBD to THC of 1:1 or higher, which means there is an equal or greater amount of CBD in the cannabis as there is of THC. The strains used for most other medical conditions, including FDA-approved Sativex® spray, is 1:1, containing equal amounts of CBD and THC. Because CBD counteracts most of the psychoactive effects of THC, these balanced medical-grade strains and extracts, in standard doses, are not associated with psychosis.

Dosing

At this time, the use of CBD for the long-term treatment of schizophrenia or any psychotic condition is not recommended. Several significant studies are ongoing, to address the possible addition of CBD to treatment with other known anti-psychotic medications. This would only be done under the very close supervision of a psychiatrist.

Dosing for an acute psychotic episode resulting from too much THC

I will say, however, that there is plenty practical, scientific and clinical evidence to support the use of CBD to treat a mild, acute episode of psychosis incurred by excessive use of cannabis/THC. CBD acts by antagonizing THC at the CB1 receptors, decreasing the effects of the THC. The recommended dose for this case would be CBD 20-60mg under the tongue one time.

Chapter 21: Neurodegenerative Diseases

Most, if not all, neurodegenerative diseases, including Alzheimer's disease, Parkinson's disease, Huntington's, and ALS, are caused by chronic inflammation in and around neurons, characterized by a loss of neurons in particular regions of the nervous system. It is believed that this nerve cell loss underlies the subsequent decline in cognitive and motor function that patients experience while suffering from these diseases. Inflammation is the common denominator among the diverse list of neurodegenerative diseases, having been implicated as a critical mechanism that is responsible for the progressive nature of neurodegeneration.

At present, there are few therapies for the wide range of neurodegenerative diseases [85]. The actual cause of the inflammation is thought to be due to chronic inflammation in response to misfolded proteins and protein plaques. The initial cause of these 'toxic' protein configurations within the neurons can be genetic, environmental, post-injury or post-infectious. However, once the protein misfolds occur, the proteins are considered foreign bodies and the immune system cascade is implemented to phagocytize the portions of the neuron that have the misfolded proteins.

The microglia and astroglia cells are the immune cells in the brain, and, like immune cells in the body, they have CB2 receptors. The chronic immune response, both cellular and pro-inflammatory chemicals, can be moderated to reduce or halt progression of the chronic inflammatory damage to these 'toxic' neurons.

Acute/Traumatic Brain Injury

Traumatic brain injury (TBI) and stroke both result in a protracted and intense localized inflammatory response in the affected area of the brain. CBD is postulated to improve the outcomes of TBI and stroke due to modulation of the often-damaging effects of the inflammatory response. Increases in brain levels of endocannabinoids following pathogenic events suggest that this system plays a role in compensatory repair mechanisms. Stroke and TBI-induced behavioral deficits, such as learning and memory, neurological motor impairments, post-traumatic convulsions or seizures, and anxiety also respond to manipulations of the endocannabinoid system.[69]

Alzheimer's, Parkinson's, and Huntington's are all neurodegenerative diseases. The dementia that occurs from repeated or severe head trauma is also a neurodegenerative condition. A neurodegenerative disease is characterized by progressive degeneration and/or death of nerve cells. Neurodegenerative diseases affect the neurons in the human brain, which are building blocks of the nervous system. Usually neurons don't replace or reproduce themselves, so when they become damaged by degeneration, it is usually permanent. As the disease progresses, problems with movement and mental functioning occur. Dementia is something caused by neurodegenerative diseases, such as Alzheimer's, and is responsible for the greatest burden associated with neurodegenerative diseases.

Alzheimer's is a neurodegenerative disease with age as the greatest risk factor. The majority of people with Alzheimer's are over the age of 65, and the risk of developing the disease doubles every 5 years after the age of 65. Family history and genetics have also been found to be risk factors. Researchers are working on finding out which factors linked to Alzheimer's development could potentially be managed. While Alzheimer's mostly impacts a person's mental functioning, Parkinson's affects their physical movement. Just as with Alzheimer's, Parkinson's generally affects people over the age of 60; Huntington's, meanwhile, is an inherited condition that can affect people of any age, with most cases occurring around 30-50 years of age.

Neurodegenerative Disease Symptoms:

- Forgetfulness
- Memory loss
- Anxiety

- Agitation
- Loss of inhibition
- Mood changes
- Apathy
- Tremors
- Slowness of movement
- Rigidity

All neurodegenerative diseases mentioned above are caused by the destructive effects of misfolded proteins inside of nerve cells. Normal proteins are the bridges and transportation system inside of the cell. The proteins are shaped in specific patterns to function correctly for this transportation goal. The proteins can become misfolded due to various reasons (genetics, oxidative stress, toxins), and this can occur in different centers of the brain. When this occurs in one center it might cause issues with memory, and in another center, it might cause a movement disorder.

These misfolded proteins don't work correctly, and they accumulate like trash inside the nerve cell. The immune system uses various means to remove the damaged proteins from the nerve cells. Often as part of this removal process, the nerve cell is damaged. If the nerve cell is damaged repeatedly or severely, it dies. This process of nerve destruction and death is very slow. It usually takes several decades from the onset of the disease until the first symptoms are obvious. Underlying all of this is the immune system in the brain causing inflammation and gradual cell death.

Unfortunately, as of now, there is no cure for these neurodegenerative conditions. There are some treatments to help manage the symptoms, but nothing yet that addresses the causes or progression of these diseases. There are many FDA-approved medications for the symptoms of these neurodegenerative conditions, but none of the available medications actually slow down or stop the formation of the misfolded proteins or the immune system gradually killing nerve cells.

CBD Treatment

CBD and cannabis have been shown in several studies to be potentially beneficial in the treatment of some symptoms caused by neurodegenerative diseases, but also it can stop or greatly decrease the underlying disease process caused by the immune system. CBD stimulates the CB2 receptors found on the immune system cells in the brain, which results in a decreased inflammatory response. Therefore, long-term use of CBD is likely to decrease the extent of damage caused by the inflammatory response.

As discussed in earlier chapters, CBD can improve symptoms of tremor, spasm, depression, anxiety, and pain that can accompany some of these conditions. In addition to potentially delaying or halting the progress of neurodegenerative diseases, CBD also can positively impact many of these symptoms.

THC stimulates the CB1 receptors found of the neurons, and this results in more decreased presence of these misfolded proteins through various cellular activities. Neurodegenerative conditions are best treated with a combination of CBD and THC.

Dosing for prevention and improvement of neurodegenerative conditions

Long-term daily use of CBD extract can have therapeutic effects on preventing the onset, halting the progression, and decreasing the symptoms of neurodegenerative conditions.

CBD EXTRACT; ADULT DOSE (NOT RECOMMENDED IN CHILDREN): 10MG OF CBD EXTRACT UNDER THE TONGUE, MORNING, AFTERNOON AND BEDTIME.

Treatment Doesn't Always Work

Medicine is an art, more than it is a science. Sometimes the recommended treatment doesn't work. It may not work because the dose wasn't correct, or it may not work because the underlying condition causing the symptoms are more severe than originally thought.

Neurodegenerative conditions follow a slow progression, so it may be difficult to judge a patient's response to a medication without close observation by a caregiver. Start out with the recommended dose and maintain it for 3-6 months to determine efficacy. If the condition continues to progress, try increasing the dose to 20mg three times a day is appropriate. Usually, it is not necessary to go to any higher dose because of the nature of this very slow, chronic disease process.

Involving Medical Professionals

Dementia and neurodegenerative diseases can cause serious and sometimes life-threatening conditions. Treatment for these conditions needs to be managed by a physician. Always involve your psychiatrist, neurologist or treating physician with decisions to add CBD or medical cannabis to the treatment of these conditions.

Chapter 22: Addiction

Addiction is a psychiatric disorder characterized by repeated, compulsive engagement in rewarding stimuli despite negative consequences; it is a chronic disease, with effects on motivation, brain reward, and memory-related bran circuitry. An individual with addiction pathologically pursues reward or relief by substance use or other behaviors. While there is a major focus on drug and alcohol addiction, addiction can come in many forms, and affects millions of Americans daily.

The group called Sober Nation explains addiction as follows: "While the degrees of separation that exist between addiction and dependence can be can vague, those who display true addictive behaviors focus their energies on obtaining the substance or performing an activity to such an absolute degree they fail to meet their personal, social, familial, educational and professional responsibilities. Additionally, those who are in the grips of addiction act impulsively and even recklessly and will continue to engage in this pattern of behavior despite the consequences of their actions."

There is no direct cause of addiction, but there are certainly a number of important risk factors, such as genetic and environmental influences, psychological history, and childhood history of abuse.

When discussing addiction, dopamine is often a point of discussion. Most addictions result, directly or indirectly, in the brain's reward system flooding the circuit with dopamine. Dopamine is a neurotransmitter, or a type of chemical that transmits signals in certain areas of the brain; dopamine works in those areas that regulate movement, motivation, emotions, and feelings of pleasure.

When a person takes drugs or participates in certain addictive behaviors, they can overstimulate this system, producing euphoric effects. These euphoric effects strongly reinforce the drug use, causing a person to repeat the behavior. What is actually happening during this process is the hippocampus (part of the brain involved with memory) is laying down memories of this rapid sense of satisfaction, causing the amygdala (part of the brain responsible for emotional responses) to create a conditioned response to the drug or behavior.

When a person repeatedly takes drugs or participates an addictive behavior, over time, their brain begins to adjust to the overwhelming surges of dopamine by producing less of the chemical or reducing the number of receptors that can receive dopamine signals. When this happens, a person needs to keep taking more of the drug or exhibiting the behavior more intensely in order to bring their dopamine function back up to normal; this is known as developing tolerance.

Examples of Addiction:

- Drug
- Alcohol
- Gambling
- Sex
- Shopping
- Exercise
- Internet
- Pornography
- Video Games
- Nicotine

Scientists have found that the symptoms of craving are mediated by increased transmission of the neurotransmitter glutamate, found in areas of the brain such as the hippocampus, the region in the brain responsible for learning and memory. This may explain why withdrawal symptoms such as anxiety, irritability, sweating, and palpitations can occur years into abstinence, when a situation or person stimulates a drug-related memory, creating a greater risk of relapse.

CBD Treatment

As was discussed earlier in the book, cannabinoid receptors are concentrated in several centers of the brain. One of those centers is the reward center, called the nucleus accumbens, which plays a significant role in addiction.

Research has shown that CBD can reduce the occurrence of ‘cue-induced cravings.” This is a craving brought on by a specific trigger, such as craving a cigarette each time you get on the phone. Once again, we see CBD impacting health by modifying the response to a stored memory in the hippocampus. CBD’s well documented effects of improving mood and reducing anxiety probably also contribute to its effects of helping with addiction recovery, discussed in other chapters.

According to an article by Yasmin L. Hurd, et al. in various studies done with animals, CBD showed positive impacts on withdrawal symptoms. It consistently decreased stress vulnerability and improved performance in numerous animal models of cognitive impairment. CBD acted as an antidepressant and decreased compulsive behavior in rodents. It was shown to prevent cocaine-induced liver damage and lessen cardiac effects. [70]

In a study of person quitting cigarette smoking, those using the CBD inhaler each time they craved a cigarette, found that they smoked 40% fewer cigarettes compared to the placebo group where there was no change. In another recent study, heroin addicts were administered a single dose of CBD over 3 consecutive days. Their propensity for craving was then tested by exposing them to opioid-related triggers. The subjects taking CBD found their cravings were lessened, an effect that lasted for 7 days after treatment.[71]

The concept of cannabis as a “gateway drug” has been debunked by the

National Academies of Medicine in 1999. To the contrary, studies from Holland suggest that legal cannabis use actually decreased the likelihood of trying cocaine and amphetamines in the first place.[72] Furthermore, a recent study of young people with mild dependency on recreational cannabis/THC showed that CBD is an effective tool to help with the cannabis craving. CBD is an antagonist of THC and blocks the euphoric effects of THC.[73]

Doses for addiction and during withdrawal

CBD Extract: Starting adult dose (not recommended in children): 10mg of CBD extract under the tongue (sublingual absorption), morning, afternoon and bedtime. May increase by 10mg every 4-5 days depending on response to the medication. Once maximum craving relief has been achieved with a certain dose, maintain that dose. Maximum daily dose 200mg.

Treatment doesn't always work

Medicine is an art, more than it is a science. Sometimes the recommended treatment doesn't work. It may not work because the dose wasn't correct, or it may not work because the underlying condition causing the symptoms is more severe than originally thought.

Start out with the recommended CBD extract dose. If the maximum doses of CBD extract isn't providing enough relief of cravings, it is time to go back to your physician for some advice.

Involving Medical Professionals

Addictions are serious conditions, and withdrawal from opioids and some other medications can have life-threatening sequelae. Beginning the withdrawal process, whether from a medication, substance or behavior, should be considered only after close discussion with your psychiatrist or primary care physician.

As is, unfortunately, usually the case, most physicians will have very little knowledge of CBD, or medical marijuana, much less their use for overcoming addiction. However, it is important to give your doctor the opportunity to assist you in controlling your symptoms.

Do not attempt to suddenly decrease or discontinue your prescription medications or illegally obtain drugs. Involve your doctor as you gradually titrate the dose of CBD, whilst making use of other addiction treatment services to control your condition.

Chapter 23:
Tapering off Opioids

Personal Story

Cynthia, a young mother in her early 30's, was a regular patient of mine. She had injured her knee while skiing with her family over Christmas; upon examination, I diagnosed her with a meniscal tear of the knee. I referred her to an Orthopedist for surgery, but I didn't hear back from her after the surgery.

Several months later, her husband came in to see me; he was tearful and depressed. He informed me that his wife had died from an unintentional opioid overdose. She had undergone knee surgery, and the surgeon had prescribed her 90 tablets of Percocet® for post-operative pain. When she was in physical therapy, the knee would flare-up, so she continued taking Percocet®. The surgeon was usually too busy to meet with her personally, so the nurse practitioner would see her instead, and kept refilling her Percocet®.

After several months, she realized that she was becoming dependent on the Percocet®, so she stopped taking it. However, her knee pain flared up while she was at work, so she went back for more Percocet® after being off them for a month. She took about 8 tablets in one day, went into respiratory arrest, and was found at home alone, dead.

This is, unfortunately, not an uncommon story; it is repeated 100+ times a day. But I have included it here because it provides some clarity to the real issues. Opioids are for short-term use after significant injury or surgery; that should be the extent of their use. Ideally within two weeks post-op, patients should be off all opioids, utilizing other means to resolve their pain, unless they have terminal cancer.

For patients with chronic pain who are prescribed opioid medications, they have to increase the regular dose to feel the same effect. In this case, Cynthia had stopped taking opioids for a month, so she was no longer tolerant to the high dose that she had been taking. Tragically, when she restarted her usual dose of opioids during a flare-up, she overdosed and died.

Introduction

There are currently an estimated 80 million chronic pain sufferers in the US, an estimated 2 million of whom are addicted to prescription opiates. Opioids include drugs such as heroin, codeine, morphine, and pain relievers such as Oxycodone®, Fentanyl® and Vicodin®. Opioids are primarily prescribed to help relieve pain by binding to opioid receptors on cells in the brain. By lowering the number of pain signals the body sends to the brain, they change how much pain the brain perceives.

They can also affect the brain's pleasure system, causing a person to feel an addictive, euphoric high. Several centers in the brain have opioid receptors, and repeated use and abuse of an opioid can change a person's brain chemistry works, leading to psychological and physical dependence on the opioid. While opioids can be very useful for people recovering from serious injuries or surgery, they should only be taken exactly as prescribed and for only as long as necessary, usually about a week or two.

The CDC recently released a report entitled "Prescribing opioids for Chronic Pain," that recommended "In general, do not prescribe opioids as the first-line treatment for chronic pain." This guideline excluded palliative or end-of-life care. It also recommended, "avoid concurrent opioid and benzodiazepine use whenever possible."[74]

Benzodiazepines, like opioids, are respiratory depressants. They work synergistically, opioids at receptors in the medulla oblongata, and benzodiazepines as CNS depressants, so that using the drugs together greatly increases the risk of overdose. However, in part due to the same aggressive pharmaceutical marketing campaigns that have created a prescription opioid epidemic, a significant proportion of chronic pain patients are still being treated with benzodiazepine medications, such as Xanax® and Klonopin®. The FDA has recently added a black box warning to address this.

This increased use of addictive and potentially life-threatening medications has been associated with a four-fold increase in the number of deaths from prescription opioids between 1999 and 2015.[75] It is not hyperbolic to say that the opioid problem in the US has reached epidemic proportions over the past 15 or so years. On average, 72 people die from opioid overdose every day; as many as two-thirds of these deaths were in patients with legal opioid prescriptions.

The over-prescribing of opioids flies in the face of many studies that have found little evidence supporting these drugs as an effective, long-term treatment for chronic pain, because of their potential for addiction, likelihood of developing a tolerance, and risk of overdose. One study of almost one million veterans found that 71% of patients who are started on opioids and maintained on them for at least 90 days will still be taking opioids three years later.[76]

Chronic pain patients are frequently denied additional prescriptions for opioids due to failed urine drug testing, most often from marijuana (THC). These patients are suddenly without prescription opioids to manage their pain, and may seek out cheaper and more accessible alternatives, such as heroin. These illicit drugs are often cut with Fentanyl®, greatly increasing the chance of unintended overdose. On top of the 72 or so people dying from legal prescription opiate overdose every day, an additional 26 people are dying from heroin overdose.[77]

In addition, a more recent study added a new issue to the prescribed opioid epidemic. It showed dramatic increases in emergency room visits for unintentional overdoses of opioids in young children, and intentional use of family member's opioids in adolescents.[78]

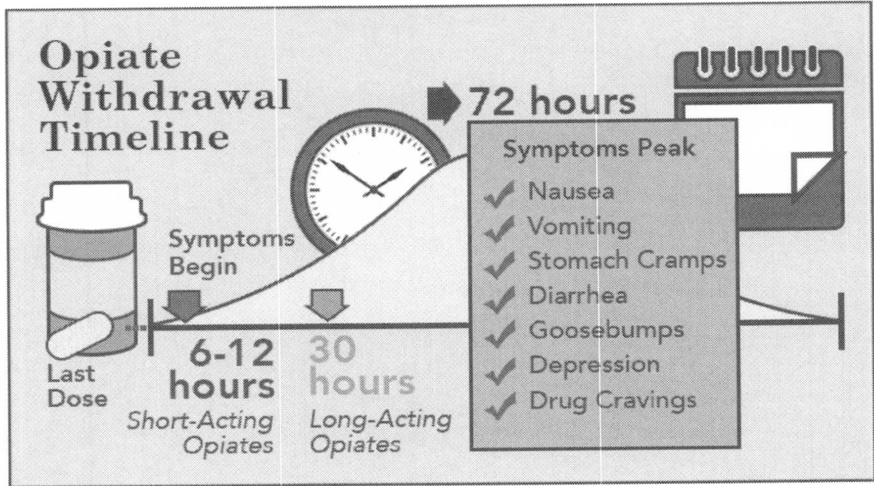

This chart from the American Addiction Center shows an opiate withdrawal timeline

When a person who is addicted to opioids stops taking them abruptly, they usually experience withdrawal. This can occur simply in between doses of opioids, or when the individual stops taking the drug altogether. Depending on how dependent a person is on opioids, the withdrawal symptoms vary from mild to severe. Early withdrawal symptoms usually start within 30 hours for long-acting opiates like Fentanyl® and OxyContin®, and within 6-12 hours for short-acting opiates, like Percocet® and Vicodin®. Late withdrawal symptoms peak within 72 hours of stopping opiates and last a week or more.

For those experiencing opioid withdrawal, there are a variety of treatment and detox options, including medical detox, which involves an individual being committed to a treatment center for 30 or more days and vital signs being monitored. There are also many treatment centers or "home-remedy" methods that take on a more natural approach treating withdrawal with dietary changes, yoga, meditation, hydration, and natural supplements.

This chapter is not about withdrawing off opioids; safe opioid withdrawal requires close medical supervision, excellent nursing, and use of several potent medications. This chapter is about gradually tapering down the opioid dose to reduce the hazards and side effects from the opioids. If this tapering is successful it can, over time, usually several months lead to the total discontinuation of the opioid medications.

CBD as an Adjunct Medication

There has been a public and political outcry in response to the dilemma of prescription opioids, as politicians' efforts over the past few years have consistently failed to mitigate the above statistics. The addition of medical cannabis or CBD may be a significant part of the solution. Cannabis was identified well over a century ago as a "tremendous success" in helping patients addicted to opioid pain medications, when, in 1889, Dr. Edward A. Birch published a seminal article of the subject. Cannabis has been shown to have efficacy in opioid sparing, as an alternative analgesic, for mood elevation and to reducing opioid withdrawal and craving.

The opioid system in the brain and ECS are parallel systems and have been shown to interact in several important ways. CB1 receptors and mu-opioid receptors (MOR) are distributed in many of the same areas of the brain, including those areas important for pain: periaqueductal gray area, ventral tegmental area, locus coeruleus, nucleus accumbens, central amygdala, prefrontal cortex, dorsal hippocampus, and medial basal hypothalamus[13] The regions of the brain that have to do with pain perception have high levels of CB1 and MOR.

Mu-opioids receptors (MOR) are similar in structure to cannabinoid receptor one (CB1) and cannabinoid receptor two (CB2). They are the site of action of innate opioids, known as endorphins, and of opioid medications.

Opioid medications reduce pain by binding to and MOR receptors in the central nervous system, leading to a decreased perception of pain via inhibition of ascending pain pathways that start in the spinal cord.

CBD externally modulates the MOR, resulting in indirect amplification of the effects of opioids at the mu-opioid binding site. This effect is associated with observed synergistic effects of CBD and opioid medications.[79] In animal models, CBD helps alleviate several symptoms of opioid withdrawal, including escape jumps, diarrhea, paw tremors and weight loss.[80, 81] CBD also improves of the affective symptoms of dysphoria and negative affect which is mediated via kapa opioid receptors (KOR).

Opioid Sparing with Cannabinoids

Opioid sparing implies that a lesser dose of opioid can be used to get the same effect through the synergistic effects of non-opioid medications. Decreasing the dose of opioids via opioid sparing leads to several harm-reduction goals, including fewer accidental overdoses and fewer adverse effects such as intractable constipation, depression and hypogonadism.

Currently, NSAIDs, antidepressants, anticonvulsants, and topical analgesic or counter-irritant preparations are being used in conjunction with opioids to reduce the amount of opioid necessary for adequate pain control. Unlike these other options for opioid sparing, however, CBD does not come with side effects. CBD, like THC, improves the efficacy of opioids on the opioid receptors in the brain; it also has a positive impact on mood, reducing anxiety commonly associated with chronic pain syndromes.[16, 68]

A recently-released analysis of the literature from the National Cannabis Industry Association (NCIA) showed that the common side-effects of chronic opioid use, including constipation, depression, hypogonadism, and nausea, were significantly reduced with concomitant use of cannabis.[82] Studies have shown that a significant percentage of patients will spontaneously discontinue opioids altogether, in lieu of CBD and other non-opioid medications.[83]

In addition to helping with opioid weaning and withdrawal, CBD has shown several therapeutic benefits with drug addiction. Substance use disorders are chronically relapsing conditions, and relapse risk persists for multiple reasons, including craving induced by drug contexts, susceptibility to stress, elevated anxiety, and impaired impulse control.

A study using an animal model of drug-seeking CBD reduced experimental anxiety, and prevented the development of high impulsivity in rats with an alcohol dependence history.[84] The results provide proof of principle supporting potential of CBD in relapse prevention.[85] Another study in the American Journal of Psychiatry used Epidiolex® (an orally administered isolate of CBD) to treat cue-related cravings and anxiety among persons with heroin use disorder; cue-craving is one of the strongest triggers for drug craving and relapse.[39]

Unfortunately, the most recent guidelines for use of medications in treatment of opioid addiction from the American Society of Addiction Medicine (2015) provides only one brief mention of medical cannabis, and provides no guidance for the use of CBD or other cannabinoid formulations, even though there are now 5 FDA-approved cannabinoid drugs.

Other opioid sparing medications

Acetaminophen, also known as Tylenol®, is one of the most commonly used over-the-counter pain medications. Unlike anti-inflammatory medications and aspirin, acetaminophen has no adverse gastrointestinal effects or untoward cardiac or kidney effects. Acetaminophen is a common opioid sparing ingredient that is combined with opioids in several common prescription medications to reduce the amount of the opiate required for pain relief; Vicodin®, Lortab®, and Oxycodone®, all contain 325 milligrams of acetaminophen as an adjunct ingredient.

Acetaminophen has been used for pain relief since it was invented one hundred years ago, but its mechanism was not understood until the past decade. Once acetaminophen is ingested, it is metabolized by the liver to a chemical called para-aminophenol, which works on pain by stimulating CB1 receptors.[86] Para-aminophenol is an inhibitor of the uptake of the naturally occurring anandamide, leading to increased levels of this endocannabinoid and increased stimulation of CB1 receptors. Para-aminophenol also stimulates TRPV1 receptors, also known as capsaicin receptors. TRPV1 is involved with the sensation of heat and sharp, burning pain.

CBD and Opioid Receptors

Opioid medications reduce pain by binding to and stimulating opioid receptors in the brain, leading to a decreased perception of pain via pain pathways that start in the spinal cord.[74] Stimulation of CB2 receptors at the site of the pain or injury results in decreased inflammation, swelling and decreased neuropathic burning pain sensation. CBD results in indirect amplification of the effects of opioids at the opioid receptor binding site.

Unfortunately, opioid receptors are heavily expressed on respiratory centers in the brainstem. Therefore, high doses of opioids can cause respiratory depression, the most common cause of opioid overdose death. There are essentially no cannabinoid receptors in the brainstem, which is the primary reason that no overdose deaths have ever been associated with cannabis use. However, although there are no fatalities associated with overdosing on cannabis, problems with decreased coordination have been associated with numerous cases of "death by accident."

How to Use Medical Cannabis for Opioid Sparing

The ideal course of treatment includes taking a dose of CBD prior to each opioid dose. When a fast-acting opioid is used, the patient will use fast-acting vaporized CBD. When a slow-release opioid is used, the patient will use CBD extract under the tongue, which comes on slowly.

For a vaporized CBD, take the recommended dose, then wait 15 minutes. The vaporized CBD will reach peak plasma concentrations in the blood in 9-23 minutes. If pain control is not sufficient, the patient will then take a second dose, again waiting 15 minutes to decide whether a before a fast-acting opioid is necessary. If there is measurable improvement in pain levels from the CBD alone, but not total pain relief, then take half of the usual dose of the fast-acting opioid medication. For example, if the usual dose is Percocet® 10/325mg, cut this in half which will give on 5mg of the active opioid ingredient, Oxycodone®. Less medication will be necessary because of the synergistic effect of CBD on opioid receptors.

The process is similar for slow-release CBD under the tongue. These CBD extracts are used to spare the use of slow-release opioids. The patient will take the dose discussed in the Flow Diagram. Wait 30 minutes, because of the slower onset of action of the extract compared to vaporized CBD. If pain relief is not sufficient, then take half the usual dose of slow-release opioid.

After 4 days at this dose of CBD, if there was insufficient pain control, increase the dose by 50%. Again, evaluate this dose for 4 days before considering increasing the dose. This is part of the slow titration of dosing with which most people will quickly become comfortable. Once pain reduction has been established with the use of CBD, the use of opioid pain medications can gradually be reduced, keeping in mind the potential for opioid withdrawal and the need for an established protocol for with your doctor for opioid weaning.

Adding Acetaminophen

As discussed above, acetaminophen decreases the perception of pain in an entirely different way via the ECS. It works by stimulating CB1 receptors in the brain, thus decreasing the perception of pain messages being sent from the spinal cord to the brain. It may also have an impact on tingling, numbness and other neuropathic pain via TRPV1 receptor activity.

The main issue with acetaminophen is that taking too much can be toxic to the liver. It is not advised to take plain acetaminophen if you are going to also take an opioid pill, since this will double the amount of acetaminophen in your system.

I recommend the 650mg slow release version of acetaminophen called Tylenol® Arthritis formula, which lasts 8 hours. The other versions of acetaminophen only last 4 - 6 hours. The maximum daily dose of acetaminophen is 3,000mg. Each opioid pill contains 325mg, and each Tylenol® Arthritis formula tablet contains 650mg. Do not exceed a total of 3,000mg in one day.

Discontinuing Opioids

If opioid sparing is successful, eventually stopping opioids altogether is the next reasonable goal. In this scenario, the goal is to replace opioids with CBD, and possibly acetaminophen. Prior to attempting this, the patient should have satisfactorily gained the skills, experience and education necessary to use CBD for opioid sparing purposes. After they have been able to successfully reduce opioid doses, many patients may attempt to taper off opioids and benzodiazepines on their own, because of the pleasant mood elevation, relief from constipation, and reduction of several opioid adverse effects. However, any tapering needs to be done in conjunction with the treating clinician to avoid serious and life-threatening opioid withdrawal or other adverse side effects.

Involving Medical Professionals

Unfortunately, most physicians will have very little knowledge of CBD, PEA or medical marijuana, and their use in chronic pain, so it is important to give your doctor the opportunity to assist you both controlling your chronic pain, and with tapering off of dangerous opioids and other medications such as Valium® or Xanax® that doctors commonly prescribe along with opioids for chronic pain. Do not attempt to suddenly decrease or discontinue your prescription medications. Involve your doctor and ask him to help you gently taper off the prescription medications while you gradually titrate the dose of CBD.

People on long-term use of opioids are typically tapered off opioid medications at a certain predetermined rate ranging from 20% to 50% per month. The medical provider should discuss the rate of tapering and expected quit date, usually from 2 to 10 months in the future. The medical provider will need to re-establish the Pain Contract with the patient with the addition of CBD, and educate the patient on the proper use, dosing, safe storage, and potential adverse effects that may be part of the sparing process. The medical provider usually monitors the progress of the tapering with regular visits and review of a pain diary.

Chapter 24: Safety & Prevention

The available evidence discussed throughout this book shows that CBD raises the cannabinoid tone in the brain and body. The main net effect of using CBD on a long-term basis as a preventive medicine, then, would be decreased inflammation in many chronic degenerative diseases that affect us as we age.

The following diseases that have been scientifically associated with chronic inflammation:

- Alzheimer's and other dementias
- Cardiovascular diseases such as heart attack and stroke
- Inflammatory-related cancers, such as bowel, prostate, breast and lung
- Autoimmune diseases, such as inflammatory arthritis, celiac disease and psoriasis

In addition, long-term improved endocannabinoid tone is associated with an improved mood, reduced anxiety and a reduction in perceived stress.[87] CBD has its therapeutic impact by raising the endocannabinoid tone throughout the brain and body, and it has been postulated that CBD can be used as preventative to decrease chronic inflammatory processes throughout various organ systems, in skin, joints and in the brain.

A recent study of 22 medical cannabis patients suffering from to a variety of conditions looked at pre- and post- brain activity and executive function after three months of medical cannabis use. Medical cannabis patients demonstrated improved task performance accompanied by changes in brain activation patterns within the cingulate cortex and frontal regions.

Interestingly, after cannabis treatment, brain activation patterns appeared more similar to those exhibited by healthy controls from previous studies than at pre-treatment, suggestive of a potential normalization of brain function relative to baseline.[88] Moreover, patients in the current study also reported improvements in clinical state and health-related measures as well as notable decreases in prescription medication use, particularly opioids and benzodiazepines after 3 months of treatment.

Safety

This book has discussed the many studies and clinical observations that confirm the safety of CBD, even for young infants. If safety were the only consideration involved, CBD extracts really could be sold next to olive oil in a grocery store. Therefore, daily use of low doses of CBD for preventive purposes is considered universally safe.

For a preventive dose, I suggest taking 25mg a day of CBD extract under the tongue or via vaporizer (10 vape inhalations a day.) This type of preventive dosing is analogous to the US Preventive Services Task Force recommendation of taking an 81mg Aspirin dose daily for prevention of cardiovascular disease and colorectal cancer.

ABBREVIATIONS

11-OH-THC- 11-Hydroxy-THC is the main active metabolite of tetrahydrocannabinol (THC) which is formed in the body after cannabis is consumed. It is more euphoric and potent than THC.

2-AG - 2-Arachidonoylglycerol is an endocannabinoid, an endogenous agonist of the CB1 receptor.

ANA- Anandamide is a fatty- acid neurotransmitter.

ASD - Autism Spectrum Disorder, describes a range of conditions classified as neurodevelopment disorders

CBC – A minor endocannabinoid with no euphoric effects. May have anti-inflammatory and antiviral effects and help to facilitate pain relief; It also may have antidepressant effects.

CBD - Cannabidiol is one of at least 144 active cannabinoids identified in cannabis. It is a major phytocannabinoid, accounting for up to 40% of the plant's extract in some strains.

CBG - Cannabigerol is a non-intoxicating cannabinoid found in the cannabis genus of plants.

CB1- The cannabinoid receptor type 1 is a G protein-coupled cannabinoid receptor located primarily in the central and peripheral nervous system.

CB2 - The cannabinoid receptor type 2 is a G protein-coupled receptor located primarily on immune system cells. It is closely related to the cannabinoid receptor type 1.

CSA- The Controlled Substances Act is the statute establishing federal US drug policy under which the manufacture, importation, possession, use, and distribution of certain substances is regulated. It was established in 1970.

FAAH- Fatty acid amide hydrolase is an enzyme. It was first shown to break down anandamide (ANA) in 1993.

FDA- The Food and Drug Administration is a federal agency of the United States Department of Health and Human Services, one of the United States federal executive departments. The FDA is responsible for protecting and promoting public health.

FM- Fibromyalgia is a medical condition characterized by chronic widespread pain and a heightened pain response to touch. Other symptoms include fatigue to a degree that normal activities are affected, sleep problems, and troubles with memory.

GRAS- Generally recognized as safe is an FDA designation that a chemical or substance added to food is considered safe by experts, and so is exempted from the usual Federal Food, Drug, and Cosmetic Act food additive tolerance requirements.

IBD- Inflammatory bowel disease is a group of inflammatory conditions of the colon and small intestine. Crohn's disease and ulcerative colitis are the principal types of inflammatory bowel disease.

IBS- Irritable bowel syndrome is a group of symptoms-including abdominal pain and changes in the pattern of bowel movements without any evidence of underlying damage.

MDD- Major depressive disorder, also known simply as depression, is a mental disorder characterized by at least two weeks of low mood that is present across most situations. It is often accompanied by low self-esteem, loss of interest in normally enjoyable activities, low energy, and pain without a clear cause.

MS- Multiple sclerosis is a demyelinating, autoimmune disease in which the insulating covers of nerve cells in the brain and spinal cord are damaged. This damage disrupts the ability of parts of the nervous system to communicate, resulting in a range of signs and symptoms, including physical, mental, and sometimes psychiatric problems.

PEA- Palmitoylethanolamide is an endogenous fatty acid amide that stimulates receptors in the brain. PEA has been demonstrated to bind to receptors inside the cell nucleus, not on the cell membrane, and exerts a great variety of biological functions similar to CBD, related to chronic pain and inflammation.

PTSD- Post-traumatic stress disorder is a severe anxiety disorder that can develop after a person is exposed to a traumatic event, such as sexual assault, warfare, traffic collisions, or other threats on a person's life.

RA- Rheumatoid arthritis is a chronic, inherited, autoimmune disorder that primarily affects joints. It typically results in warm, swollen, and painful joints that can become disfigured in more severe cases.

RSHO- Real Scientific Hemp Oil is A brand of hemp oil that is high in CBD. It is not to be confused with Rick Simpson Oil (RSO), a very potent THC-rich oil for late stage cancer.

RSO- Rick Simpson oil, also known as Phoenix Tears. This is a very potent, THC-rich oil, used in a 90-day regimen for late stage cancer. Requires a physician's supervision.

THC- Tetrahydrocannabinol refers to a psychotropic cannabinoid and is the principal psychoactive constituent of cannabis.

TRPV1- The transient receptor potential cation channel subfamily V member 1, also known as the capsaicin receptor and the vanilloid receptor 1. It is a receptor that is important for temperature regulation and sensation of heat.

INDEX

REFERENCES

1 Evanoff, A.B., et al., Physicians-in-training are not prepared to prescribe medical marijuana. Drug Alcohol Depend, 2017. 180: p. 151-5.

2 Front Matter | The Health Effects of Cannabis and Cannabinoids: The Current State of Evidence and Recommendations for Research | The National Academies Press. 2019.

3 Tóth, K.F., et al., Cannabinoid Signaling in the Skin: Therapeutic Potential of the "C(ut)annabinoid" System, in Molecules. 2019.

4 Zou, S. and U. Kumar, Cannabinoid Receptors and the Endocannabinoid System: Signaling and Function in the Central Nervous System. Int J Mol Sci, 2018. 19(3).

5 Mattes, R.D.e.a., Bypassing the first-pass effect for the therapeutic use of cannabinoids. Pharmacology Biochemistry and Behavior, 1993. 44(3).

6 Conte, R., et al., Recent Advances in Nanoparticle-Mediated Delivery of Anti-Inflammatory Phytocompounds. Int J Mol Sci, 2017. 18(4).

7 Bonn-Miller, M.O., et al., Labeling Accuracy of Cannabidiol Extracts Sold Online, in JAMA. 2017. p. 1708-9.

8 Vandrey, R.e.a., Cannabinoid Dose and Label Accuracy in Edible Medical Cannabis Products. JAMA, 2019. 313(24): p. 2491-2493.

9 Hemp CBD Infused Product Market Projected to Triple by 2022. 2019.

10 Russo, E.B., Taming THC: potential cannabis synergy and phytocannabinoid-terpenoid entourage effects. Br J Pharmacol, 2011. 163(7): p. 1344-64.

11 Bolognini, D., Pharmacological properties of the phytocannabinoids Δ9-tetrahydrocannabivarin and cannabidiol. 2010.

12 Evanoff, A.B.e.a., Physicians-in-training are not prepared to prescribe medical marijuana. Drug and Alcohol Dependency, 2017. 180.

13 Ujváry, I. and L. Hanuš, Human Metabolites of Cannabidiol: A Review on Their Formation, Biological Activity, and Relevance in Therapy. Cannabis Cannabinoid Res, 2016. 1(1): p. 90-101.

14 Iffland, K. and F. Grotenhermen, An Update on Safety and Side Effects of Cannabidiol: A Review of Clinical Data and Relevant Animal Studies. Cannabis Cannabinoid Res, 2017. 2(1): p. 139-154.

15 M, B., 14% of Americans Say They Use CBD Products. Galllup, 2019.

16 Azer V, B.J., Charles AM et al, Collective View of CBD. Cowen Outperform, 2019.

17 Zynerba Pharmaceuticals Announces Positive Top Line Results in ZYN002 Open Label Phase 2 FAB-C Study in Children with Fragile X Syndrome - Zynerba. 2017 2017-09-28; Available from: http://zynerba.com/zynerba-pharmaceuticals-announces-positive-top-line-results-zyn002-open-label-phase-2-fab-c-study-children-fragile-x-syndrome/.

18 Pertwee, R.G., The diverse CB1 and CB2 receptor pharmacology of three plant cannabinoids: Δ9-tetrahydrocannabinol, cannabidiol and Δ9-tetrahydrocannabivarin. Br J Pharmacol, 2008. 153(2): p. 199-215.

19 Organization, W.H., Cannabidol (CBD) Pre-Review Report - WHO Expert Committee on Drug Dependence. 2017, World Health Organization (WHO): Geneva.

20 Kaplan, B.L.F., A.E.B. Springs, and N.E. Kaminski, The Profile of Immune Modulation by Cannabidiol (CBD) Involves Deregulation of Nuclear Factor of Activated T Cells (NFAT). Biochem Pharmacol, 2008. 76(6): p. 726-37.

21 Koppel, B.S., et al., Systematic review: Efficacy and safety of medical marijuana in selected neurologic disorders: Report of the Guideline Development Subcommittee of the American Academy of Neurology. Neurology, 2014. 82(17): p. 1556-63.

22 Abrams, D.I., et al., Cannabis in painful HIV-associated sensory neuropathy: a randomized placebo-controlled trial. Neurology, 2007. 68(7): p. 515-21.

23 Russo, E.B., Cannabinoids in the management of difficult to treat pain. Ther Clin Risk Manag, 2008. 4(1): p. 245-59.

24 Hammell, D., et al., Transdermal cannabidiol reduces inflammation and pain-related behaviours in a rat model of arthritis. Eur J Pain, 2016. 20(6): p. 936-48.

25 Piper, B.J., et al., Substitution of medical cannabis for pharmaceutical agents for pain, anxiety, and sleep. J Psychopharmacol, 2017. 31(5): p. 569-575.

26 Antonaci, F., et al., Recent advances in migraine therapy. Springerplus, 2016. 5: p. 637.

27 Pascual, J., R. Colas, and J. Castillo, Epidemiology of chronic daily headache. Curr Pain Headache Rep, 2001. 5(6): p. 529-36.

28 Russo, E.B., Clinical endocannabinoid deficiency (CECD): can this concept explain therapeutic benefits of cannabis in migraine, fibromyalgia, irritable bowel syndrome and other treatment-resistant conditions? Neuro Endocrinol Lett, 2004. 25(1-2): p. 31-9.

29 Baron, E.P., Comprehensive Review of Medicinal Marijuana, Cannabinoids, and Therapeutic Implications in Medicine and

Headache: What a Long Strange Trip It's Been. Headache, 2015. 55(6): p. 885-916.

30 O'Shaughnessy. Cannabinoids for Prevention of Migraines. 2017; Available from: http://www.beyondthc.com/cannabinoids-for-prevention-of-migraines/.

31 Camilleri, M., et al., Cannabinoid receptor 1 gene and irritable bowel syndrome: phenotype and quantitative traits, in Am J Physiol Gastrointest Liver Physiol. 2013. p. G553-60.

32 De Filippis, D., et al., Cannabidiol Reduces Intestinal Inflammation through the Control of Neuroimmune Axis, in PLoS One. 2011.

33 Gui, H., et al., Expression of cannabinoid receptor 2 and its inhibitory effects on synovial fibroblasts in rheumatoid arthritis. Rheumatology, 2019. 53(5): p. 802-809.

34 Malfait, A.M., et al., The nonpsychoactive cannabis constituent cannabidiol is an oral anti-arthritic therapeutic in murine collagen-induced arthritis. Proc Natl Acad Sci U S A, 2000. 97(17): p. 9561-6.

35 Ständer, S.e.a., Distribution of cannabinoid receptor 1 (CB1) and 2 (CB2) on sensory nerve fibers and adnexal structures in human skin. Journal of Dermatological Science, 2005. 38(3): p. 177-188.

36 Stander, S., H.W. Reinhardt, and T.A. Luger, [Topical cannabinoid agonists. An effective new possibility for treating chronic pruritus]. Hautarzt, 2006. 57(9): p. 801-7.

37 Olah, A., et al., Cannabidiol exerts sebostatic and antiinflammatory effects on human sebocytes. J Clin Invest, 2014. 124(9): p. 3713-24.

38 Sekar, K. and A. Pack, Epidiolex as adjunct therapy for treatment of refractory epilepsy: a comprehensive review with a focus on adverse effects. F1000Res, 2019. 8.

39 Summary, M., Epidiolex (cannabidiol) dosing, indications, interactions, adverse effects, and more. Medscape, 2019.

40 Rosenberg, E.C., P.H. Patra, and B.J. Whalley, Therapeutic effects of cannabinoids in animal models of seizures, epilepsy, epileptogenesis, and epilepsy-related neuroprotection. Epilepsy Behav, 2017. 70(Pt B): p. 319-327.

41 Rosenberg, E.C., et al., Cannabinoids and Epilepsy. Neurotherapeutics, 2015. 12(4): p. 747-68.

42 Jones, N.A., et al., Cannabidiol exerts anti-convulsant effects in animal models of temporal lobe and partial seizures. Seizure, 2012. 21(5): p. 344-52.

43 Perucca, E., Cannabinoids in the Treatment of Epilepsy: Hard Evidence at Last? J Epilepsy Res, 2017. 7(2): p. 61-76.

44 Szaflarski, J.P., et al., Long-term safety and treatment effects of cannabidiol in children and adults with treatment-resistant epilepsies: Expanded access program results. Epilepsia, 2018. 59(8): p. 1540-1548.

45 DeLorenzo, R.J., Marijuana and its receptor protein in brain control epilepsy. 2019.

46 Fiz, J., et al., Cannabis Use in Patients with Fibromyalgia: Effect on Symptoms Relief and Health-Related Quality of Life. PLoS One, 2011. 6(4).

47 Vermersch, P. and M. Trojano, Tetrahydrocannabinol:Cannabidiol Oromucosal Spray for Multiple Sclerosis-Related Resistant Spasticity in Daily Practice. European Neurology, 2019. 76(5-6): p. 216-226.

48 Giacoppo, S., et al., A new formulation of cannabidiol in cream shows therapeutic effects in a mouse model of experimental autoimmune encephalomyelitis, in Daru. 2015.

49 Massi, P., et al., Cannabidiol as potential anticancer drug. Br J Clin Pharmacol, 2013. 75(2): p. 303-12.

50 Ligresti, A.e.a., Antitumor Activity of Plant Cannabinoids with Emphasis on the Effect of Cannabidiol on Human Breast Carcinoma. The Journal of Pharmacological and Experimental Therapeutics, 2019.

51 Cordon-Cardo, C. and C. Prives, At the Crossroads of Inflammation and Tumorigenesis. 1999.

52 Zanelati, T.V., et al., Antidepressant-like effects of cannabidiol in mice: possible involvement of 5-HT1A receptors. Br J Pharmacol, 2010. 159(1): p. 122-8.

53 Sales, A.J., et al., Antidepressant-like effect induced by Cannabidiol is dependent on brain serotonin levels. Prog Neuropsychopharmacol Biol Psychiatry, 2018. 86: p. 255-261.

54 Shoval, G., et al., Prohedonic Effect of Cannabidiol in a Rat Model of Depression. Neuropsychobiology, 2019. 73(2): p. 123-129.

55 Babson, K.A., J. Sottile, and D. Morabito, Cannabis, Cannabinoids, and Sleep: a Review of the Literature. Curr Psychiatry Rep, 2017. 19(4): p. 23.

56 Lintzeris, N., et al., Nabiximols for the Treatment of Cannabis Dependence: A Randomized Clinical Trial. JAMA Internal Medicine, 2019. 179(9): p. 1242-1253.

57 Bandelow, B. and S. Michaelis, Epidemiology of anxiety disorders in the 21st century. Dialogues Clin Neurosci, 2015. 17(3): p. 327-35.

58 Abrams, D.I., The therapeutic effects of Cannabis and cannabinoids: An update from the National Academies of Sciences, Engineering and Medicine report. Eur J Intern Med, 2018.

59 Blanco, C., Pharmacotherapy of social anxiety disorder. Biological Psychiatry, 2002. 51(1): p. 109-120.

60 Blessing, E.M., et al., Cannabidiol as a Potential Treatment for Anxiety Disorders. Neurotherapeutics, 2015. 12(4): p. 825-36.

61 de Mello Schier, A.R., et al., Antidepressant-like and anxiolytic-like effects of cannabidiol: a chemical compound of Cannabis sativa. CNS Neurol Disord Drug Targets, 2014. 13(6): p. 953-60.

62 Nardo M, C.P., Gomes FV, et al, Cannabidiol reverses the mCPP□induced increase in marble□burying behavior - Nardo - 2014 - Fundamental & Clinical Pharmacology - Wiley Online Library. Fundamental and Clinical Pharmacology, 2013.

63 Poleg, S., et al., Cannabidiol as a suggested candidate for treatment of autism spectrum disorder. Prog Neuropsychopharmacol Biol Psychiatry, 2019. 89: p. 90-96.

64 Aran, A., et al., Brief Report: Cannabidiol-Rich Cannabis in Children with Autism Spectrum Disorder and Severe Behavioral Problems-A Retrospective Feasibility Study. J Autism Dev Disord, 2019. 49(3): p. 1284-1288.

65 Bonaccorso, S., et al., Cannabidiol (CBD) use in psychiatric disorders: A systematic review. Neurotoxicology, 2019. 74: p. 282-298.

66 Zuardi, A., et al., Cannabidiol for the treatment of psychosis in Parkinson's disease:. http://dx.doi.org/10.1177/0269881108096519, 2008.

67 Zuardi, A.W., et al., Cannabidiol monotherapy for treatment-resistant schizophrenia:. http://dx.doi.org/10.1177/0269881106060967, 2006.

68 Englund, A., et al., Cannabidiol inhibits THC-elicited paranoid symptoms and hippocampal-dependent memory impairment:. http://dx.doi.org/10.1177/0269881112460109, 2012.

69 Hayakawa, K., K. Mishima, and M. Fujiwara, Therapeutic Potential of Non-Psychotropic Cannabidiol in Ischemic Stroke. Pharmaceuticals, 2010. 3(7): p. 2197-2212.

70 Hurd, Y.L., et al., Early Phase in the Development of Cannabidiol as a Treatment for Addiction: Opioid Relapse Takes Initial Center Stage. Neurotherapeutics, 2015. 12(4): p. 807-15.

71 Hurd, Y.L., et al., Cannabidiol for the Reduction of Cue-Induced Craving and Anxiety in Drug-Abstinent Individuals With Heroin Use Disorder: A Double-Blind Randomized Placebo-Controlled Trial. https://doi.org/10.1176/appi.ajp.2019.18101191, 2019.

72 Watson, S.J., J.A. Benson, Jr., and J.E. Joy, Marijuana and medicine: assessing the science base: a summary of the 1999 Institute of Medicine report. Arch Gen Psychiatry, 2000. 57(6): p. 547-52.

73 Bhattacharyya, S., et al., Opposite effects of delta-9-tetrahydrocannabinol and cannabidiol on human brain function and psychopathology. Neuropsychopharmacology, 2010. 35(3): p. 764-74.

74 Chapman, C.R., et al., Opioid pharmacotherapy for chronic non-cancer pain in the United States: a research guideline for developing an evidence-base. J Pain, 2010. 11(9): p. 807-29.

75 Ling, W., L. Mooney, and M. Hillhouse, Prescription opioid abuse, pain and addiction: Clinical issues and implications. Drug Alcohol Rev, 2011. 30(3): p. 300-5.

76 Hayes, C.J., et al., Health-Related Quality of Life among Chronic Opioid Users, Nonchronic Opioid Users, and Nonopioid Users with Chronic Noncancer Pain. Health Serv Res, 2018.

77 Abuse, N.I.o.D., Trends & Statistics. 2017, NIDA.

78 Elzey, M.J., S.M. Barden, and E.S. Edwards, Patient Characteristics and Outcomes in Unintentional, Non-fatal Prescription Opioid Overdoses: A Systematic Review. Pain Physician, 2016. 19(4): p. 215-28.

77 Abuse, N.I.o.D., Trends & Statistics. 2017, NIDA.

78 Elzey, M.J., S.M. Barden, and E.S. Edwards, Patient Characteristics and Outcomes in Unintentional, Non-fatal Prescription Opioid Overdoses: A Systematic Review. Pain Physician, 2016. 19(4): p. 215-28.

79 Cooper, Z.D., et al., Impact of co-administration of oxycodone and smoked cannabis on analgesia and abuse liability. Neuropsychopharmacology, 2018.

80 Neelakantan, H., et al., Distinct interactions of cannabidiol and morphine in three nociceptive behavioral models in mice. Behav

81 Prud'homme, M., R. Cata, and D. Jutras-Aswad, Cannabidiol as an Intervention for Addictive Behaviors: A Systematic Review of the Evidence. Subst Abuse, 2015. 9: p. 33-8.

82 Nielsen, S., et al., Opioid-Sparing Effect of Cannabinoids: A Systematic Review and Meta-Analysis. Neuropsychopharmacology, 2017. 42(9): p. 1752-65.

83 Khan, S.P., T.A. Pickens, and D.J. Berlau, Perspectives on cannabis as a substitute for opioid analgesics. Pain Manag, 2019. 9(2): p. 191-203.

84 Gonzalez-Cuevas, G., et al., Unique treatment potential of cannabidiol for the prevention of relapse to drug use: preclinical proof of principle. Neuropsychopharmacology, 2018. 43(10): p. 2036-45.

85 de Carvalho, C.R. and R.N. Takahashi, Cannabidiol disrupts the reconsolidation of contextual drug-associated memories in Wistar rats. Addict Biol, 2017. 22(3): p. 742-751.

86 Brune, K., B. Renner, and G. Tiegs, Acetaminophen/paracetamol: A history of errors, failures and false decisions. Eur J Pain, 2015. 19(7): p. 953-65.

87 Patel, S. and C.J. Hillard, Role of Endocannabinoid Signaling in Anxiety and Depression. Curr Top Behav Neurosci, 2009. 1.

88 Gruber, S.A., et al., The Grass Might Be Greener: Medical Marijuana Patients Exhibit Altered Brain Activity and Improved Executive Function after 3 Months of Treatment. Front Pharmacol, 2017. 8.

Made in the USA
Columbia, SC
25 March 2020

90002697R00126